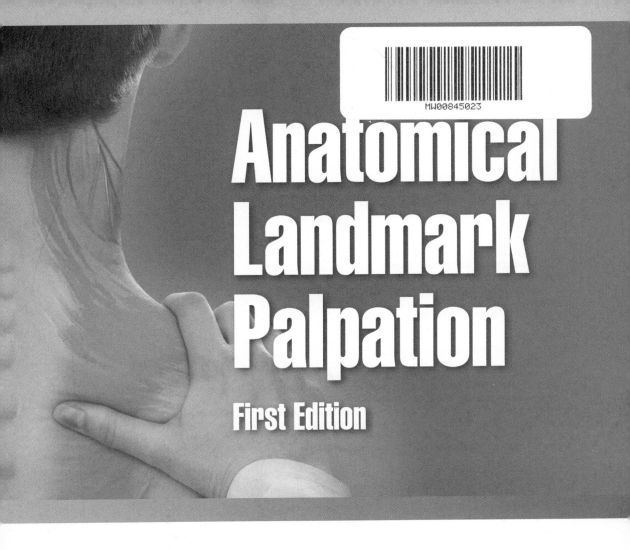

Anatomical Landmark Palpation

First Edition

Paula J. Maxwell, PhD, ATC

Interim Associate Dean
James Madison University
College of Health and Behavioral Studies
Harrisonburg, Virginia

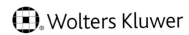 Wolters Kluwer

Philadelphia • Baltimore • New York • London
Buenos Aires • Hong Kong • Sydney • Tokyo

Senior Acquisitions Editor: Emily Lupash
Product Development Editor: John Larkin
Product Production Manager: David Saltzberg
Marketing Manager: Shauna Kelley
Designer: Stephen Druding
Compositor: Absolute Service, Inc.

LWW.com

*To my Mom, whose parenting style
provided me with the confidence to try
new things and taught me that the only
things in which I could succeed were
those things I was courageous enough
to attempt. Thanks for all my successes!
Mom, I know you love me dearly
and are profoundly proud of me.
Thanks for loving me, believing in me,
and encouraging me in every step of life.
I know it's hard that life's details are
slowly slipping away, but please know
I'm walking beside you, holding your
hand, and protecting the memories for
both of us.*

Preface

My former athletic training and physical therapy students spearheaded the need for this palpation project. As I was teaching them in classroom and laboratory settings, they requested a resource that would allow them to review palpations outside of the formal educational setting. Students found they wanted to review palpation techniques throughout their curriculum but didn't have a resource that would allow them to do that, especially a resource that "showed" them (i.e., walked them through the steps in a video format) how to perform the palpations. Also, as a practicing clinician, I realized that I and many of my colleagues were not as proficient as we could be in specific palpation techniques. At that time, I started to hone my own skills in this area and soon realized this project could be a resource that could meet the needs of students and professionals alike.

The project is intended to be a supplemental resource for students in athletic training, physical therapy, occupational therapy, and other health related clinical professional programs. These videos provide the options of viewing suggested patient positioning for the palpation, skeletal and anatomical characterizations of each landmark, demonstration of the palpation from the evaluator's view and, in many cases, a side view and special tips for the locating the landmark. The web-based version also provides quiz questions for each landmark to reinforce the viewer's knowledge.

The textbook is provided as an ancillary to the web-based videos for those viewers wanting to access the information when internet is not available or is not convenient, such as when the student is in the clinical setting yet has the opportunity to review clinical information.

Both the video and the textbook provide step-by-step instructions for finding each landmark. These skills will be most helpful in courses that focus on orthopedic assessment or manual therapy techniques.

Online Videos

The online videos provide visual demonstration of the palpation of nearly 200 common bony and soft tissue landmarks in the body. Written text and audio narration accompany each video. For each landmark, the viewer is provided with several options from which to select, or the viewer can simply progress through each option in successive fashion. Viewers can select which portion of the videos they wish to view and can skip over the aspects that do not interest them or are not necessary for their study needs (e.g., a viewer may not need to review patient positioning so may only select the tip for verifying that they are on the correct landmark).

Options available for each palpation are as follows:

1) Patient positioning—The palpation is shown from a distance so patient and evaluator positioning can be observed. Though multiple patient positioning options may be available, the video depicts one of the most commonly used positions.

2) Skeletal and anatomical overlays—The landmark is identified three ways: on the skeleton only, on the anatomical body only, then the two are overlaid on each other with a fade-in/fade-out option. This latter option allows the viewer to drag the scrubber back and forth causing the skeletal and anatomical landmarks to fade-in and fade-out over each other to better understand the exact location of the landmark. Project reviewers appreciated this fade-in/fade-out function the most.

3) Palpation example—A close-up demonstration of each palpation is provided from one or more viewpoints: evaluator's view, side view, or alternate view/method. The various viewpoints are often helpful when learning the palpation.

4) Tips—When possible, special tips are provided for locating the landmark or verifying you are on the correct landmark.

5) Quiz questions—Each landmark has at least two quiz questions to help students review and reinforce their knowledge about the landmark or its palpation.

Access to the online videos is available at http://thepoint.lww.com/Maxwell1e. This website is mobile-friendly for access anytime, anywhere for your study needs. Your individual password can be accessed by using the scratch-off access code located inside the front cover of the textbook.

Acknowledgments

Special thanks for this project go to the following individuals:

Thom Slomka: Thom, thanks for not allowing me to "just borrow a video camera for an afternoon." Your vision for what this project could be and the hundreds of hours (literally) you and your staff put in to see it come to fruition were instrumental in the final project. Also, thank you for the many, many laughs we experienced throughout the project. Your sense of humor got us through the frustrations we encountered. Thank you from the depths of my heart. I owe this project to you!

University at Buffalo: This project was made possible in the early stages by an Educational Technology grant provided by the University at Buffalo. Thank you, UB, for seeing the potential in this idea and being willing to support it financially and through staff support. Special thanks also go to Martha Greatrix, Larry Scott, John Wild, and the graduate assistants for your videography assistance in the early stages of this project.

Stephanie (Kreutter) Pritchard: Your skill and attention to detail in creating the graphic overlays were remarkable. Thank you for your time and dedication to help get it right and for not settling for "good enough." Your creations are still some of my favorite parts of this project.

Liz Lyon: Thank you for the hundreds of hours you put in processing video segments. I appreciated your sense of humor, especially the times when you were viewing some of these clips in the open lab, causing people to wonder (and sometimes worry about) what you could be working on!

Jo Gundrum: Thank you for being willing to learn the processing steps then working so diligently for me in the end stages of this project. Your support means a lot. I could not have finished this project without your help!

Models and Palpators: You were key to the completion of this project! You all were wonderful (and many times very patient as we struggled with lighting or other issues). You helped make this project fun to create! Thanks for being so willing to donate your appendages for me to videotape or for being willing to palpate over and over and over again until we got it right. (Jen Stachura, I laugh with you every time I hear myself say "just one more time!")

Individual thanks go to the following models and palpators:

Sophia Bonadies	Andrew Keane	Michael Selby
Amanda Clark	Barbara Long	Maggie Smith
Tim Cuddeback	Jared Miller	Jen Stachura
Patrick Deal	Connie Peterson	Jeremie Stearns
Lisa Friesen	Elise Sawtelle	Ashley Stewart
Tim James	Shaun Scissom	John Ward

D. Lee Beard and the James Madison University Center for Instructional Technology/ Media Production staff (Dave Stoops and Ashley Caudill): Thank you for allowing me to use the studio for recordings and for assisting with the setup each time. You run a quality show!

Barbara Long: Thank you for your belief in me and in this project. Your words of encouragement, assistance with portions of the project, excitement over the final product, and your friendship in general have been greatly appreciated and have motivated me.

Louise Gilchrist: Thank you for inviting me to conduct labs for your physical therapy students—that is what started the idea of this project in the first place. Thanks also for the years of encouragement, friendship, and vision for what could be done with this project once it was complete. I'm still going to take you up on some of the research projects we discussed way back when!

Wolters Kluwer: Thank you for believing in this project and tackling some of the technology pieces that eluded us near the end. Your support and work on this project are greatly appreciated.

User's Guide/Introduction

General Palpation Instructions:

When palpating, position the patient in a comfortable position that allows you to gain clear access to the landmark of interest. Whenever possible, it is best to remove clothing from the area for unobstructed palpations.

Position yourself in a biomechanically appropriate position so you do not injure yourself during the palpation (e.g., bending rather than sitting on a stool has the potential to strain the back). Also position yourself in a way that you can visualize the landmark as well as watch the patient's face to see expressions of pain or apprehension.

Using either the thumb or the fingers, start away from the site of pain and slowly work toward the painful area. If using the thumb, use extra care because additional pressure is sometimes inadvertently applied when the thumbs are used. Palpate with confidence while continually communicating with the patient and making eye contact. Once the painful area is located, the specific landmark involved can be determined.

Directional Terms:

Remember, when following instructions for the forearm and hand/wrist, medial and lateral directions are according to anatomical position. Thus, when the arm is pronated and it is stated to move medially, the palpator should move toward the pinky side of the arm. If moving laterally, the palpator would move toward the thumb side of the arm. This reference can be confusing and will result in the wrong structures being palpated if the directions are reversed.

Confirming Muscle Palpations:

For muscle palpations, when possible (i.e. the patient is able to perform the motions/contractions), ask the patient to contract the muscle against slight resistance. This action will cause the muscle to "belly up" or contract and become more prominent for your palpation. In addition, it is often helpful to confirm the identity of the muscles or other structures surrounding the muscle of interest. To confirm the nearby muscles' identity, ask the patient to perform the motions of those muscles while palpating them. Feel for the contraction of the muscles as the patient completes the designated motion.

Contents

Contents

Preface

Acknowledgments

SECTION I · UPPER BODY PALPATIONS

SECTION II · LOWER BODY PALPATIONS

SECTION I

Upper Body
Palpations

Angle of the Jaw

Skeletal and Anatomical Landmarks

Skeletal

Anatomical

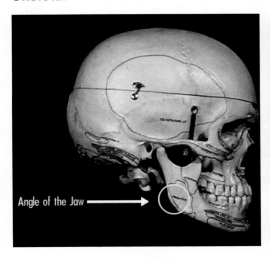

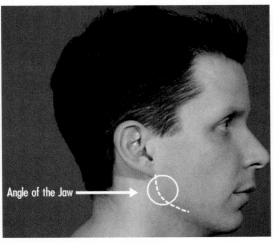

The angle of the jaw is the posterior aspect of the jaw, approximately 2–3 inches inferior to the temporomandibular joint or 1–2 inches from the earlobe.

Palpation Example

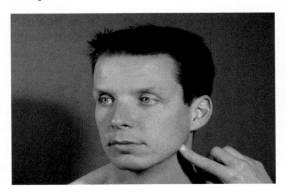

To palpate the angle of the jaw,
1) Place the patient in a seated position at the end of the treatment table. Stand in front of the patient.
2) Locate the edge of the jaw near the earlobe, then follow the jaw inferiorly and anteriorly 1–2 inches.
3) The bone turns at an 80–90 degree angle. That turn is the angle of the jaw.

◉ C1 Transverse Process

Skeletal and Anatomical Landmarks

Skeletal   **Anatomical**

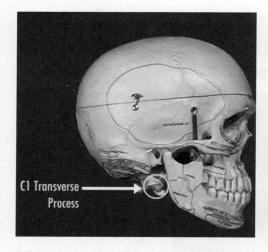
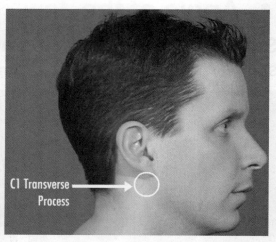

The C1 transverse process is the only palpable cervical transverse process. It lies just posterior to the angle of the jaw and just inferior to the earlobe.

Palpation Example

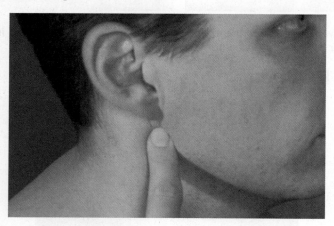

To palpate the C1 transverse process,
1) Place the patient in a seated position at the end of the treatment table. Stand facing the patient.
2) Place your finger in the groove of the neck just below the earlobe and behind the angle of the jaw.
3) Move your finger about ½–1 finger width inferiorly and gently apply inward pressure in small circular motions.
4) The transverse process will be felt as a small ball.

◉ C7 Spinous Process

Skeletal and Anatomical Landmarks

Skeletal　　　　　　　　　　　**Anatomical**

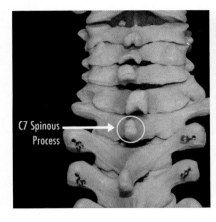

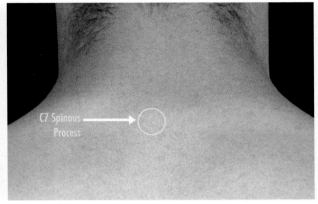

The C7 spinous process is the most prominent cervical spinous process. It is located at the base of the neck.

Palpation Example

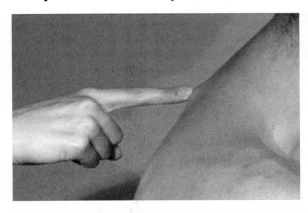

To palpate the C7 spinous process,
1) Place the patient in a seated position at the end of the treatment table. Stand to the side of the patient.
2) Ask the patient to flex the neck.
3) Locate the most prominent vertebral spinous protrusion at the base of the neck.

TIP

Flex Neck

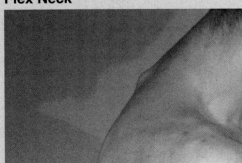

The process becomes more prominent when the patient flexes the neck.

Carotid Pulse

Skeletal and Anatomical Landmarks

Skeletal   **Anatomical**

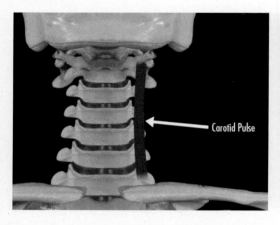

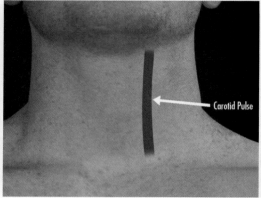

The carotid pulse is located in the groove that is formed between the thyroid cartilage and the sternocleidomastoid muscle.

Palpation Example

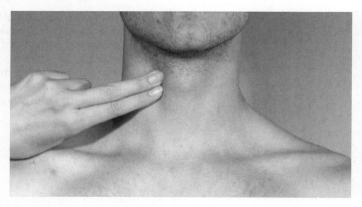

To palpate the carotid pulse,
1) Place the patient in a seated position at the end of the treatment table. Stand in front or to the side of the patient.
2) Place your index and middle fingers on the thyroid cartilage, then
3) Slide them laterally until you feel the groove between the thyroid cartilage and the sternocleido-mastoid muscle.
4) You may have to press in gently to feel the pulse.

Cricoid Rings

Skeletal and Anatomical Landmarks

Skeletal   **Anatomical**

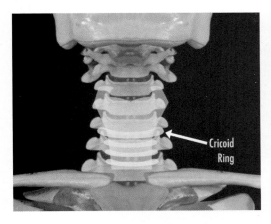

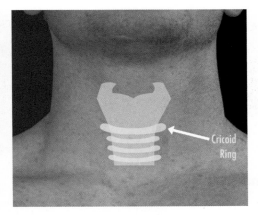

The first cricoid ring is found just below the thyroid cartilage.

Palpation Example

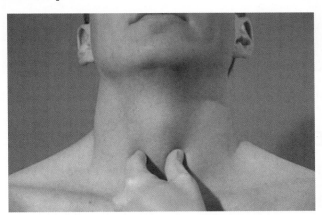

To palpate the first cricoid ring,
1) Place the patient in a seated position at the end of the treatment table. Stand in front of the patient.
2) First locate the prominent upper lip of the thyroid cartilage (known as the "Adam's Apple") then move inferiorly until the inferior edge of the thyroid cartilage is felt, about 1–2 finger widths.
3) Move slightly inferiorly to the cricoid cartilage, which will be felt as a solid ring that encircles the throat.
4) Palpate the cricoid rings with one digit or by gently grasping the lateral edges between the fingers and thumb.
5) Palpate gently to avoid invoking a gag response or injuring the area.

Hyoid

Skeletal and Anatomical Landmarks

Skeletal

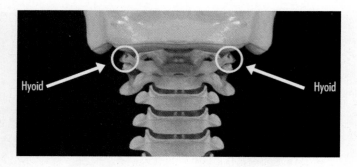

Anatomical

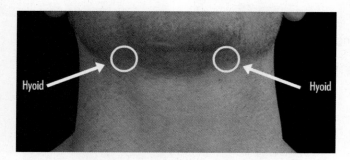

The hyoid bone is a horseshoe-shaped bone that lies just below the jaw and just above the thyroid cartilage.

Palpation Example

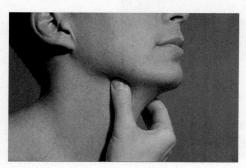

To palpate the hyoid,
1) Place the patient in a seated position at the end of the treatment table.
2) Gently place your hand around the front of the neck, under the jaw and distal to the angle of the jaw.
3) With your thumb on one side and index finger on the other, slide your hand forward as necessary until you feel small balls (which are the ends of the hyoid bone).
4) Apply gentle inward pressure while making small circular motions to best feel the hyoid.

TIP

Swallow
Asking the person to swallow will move the hyoid under your fingers, verifying the correct palpation.

Glide Side to Side
Once the hyoid is found, you can feel the bone glide side to side when applying lateral pressure.

Lacrimal Bone

Skeletal and Anatomical Landmarks

Skeletal

Anatomical

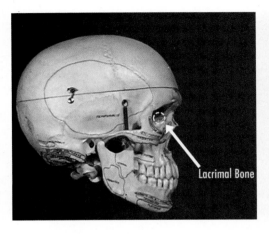 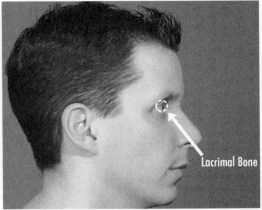

The lacrimal bone is the bone on the medial aspect of the eye near the tear duct.

Palpation Example

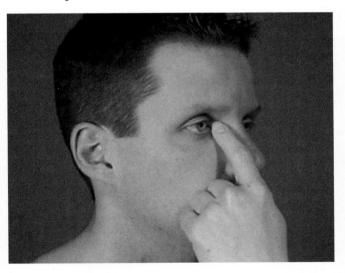

To palpate the lacrimal bone,
1) Place the patient in a seated position at the end of the treatment table.
2) Using your index finger, locate the bone on the medial aspect of the eye near the tear duct.
3) The evaluator should use a gloved hand for this palpation.

◉ Mandible

Skeletal and Anatomical Landmarks

Skeletal   **Anatomical**

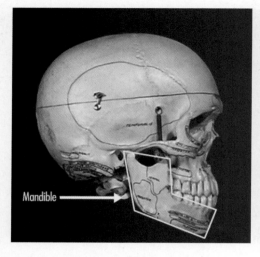 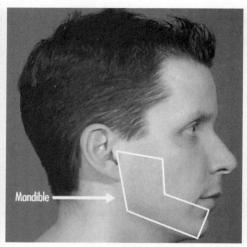

The mandible is the jaw bone.

Palpation Example

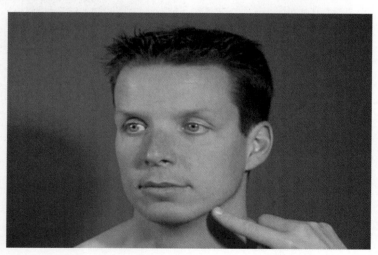

To palpate the mandible,
1) Place the patient in a seated position at the end of the treatment table.
2) Locate the jaw bone.
3) Using your fingers, palpate the full length of the jaw (mandible) from the tragus of the ear to the tip of the chin.
4) One hand may be used to stabilize the head while the other hand is used to palpate.

● Mastoid Process

Skeletal and Anatomical Landmarks

Skeletal

Anatomical

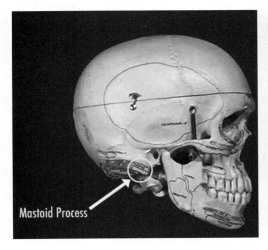

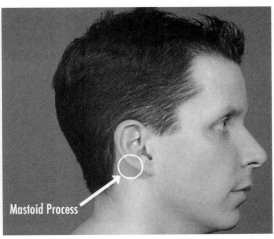

The mastoid process is the part of the occipital bone that lies behind the ear.

Palpation Example

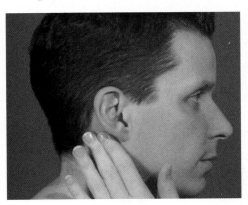

To palpate the mastoid process,
1) Place the patient in a seated position at the end of the treatment table.
2) Reach behind the ear and locate the ball-like protrusion of the skull that lies posterior to the inferior aspect of the ear.
3) Move your finger in a circular pattern on the protrusion to palpate the full structure.
4) Palpating both sides simultaneously helps stabilize the head.

Posterior View

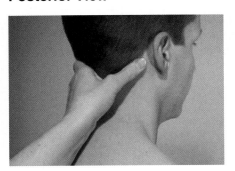

To palpate the mastoid process, locate the ball-like protrusion just posterior to the ear.

◉ Maxilla

Skeletal and Anatomical Landmarks

Skeletal   **Anatomical**

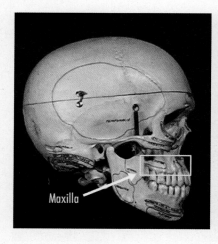 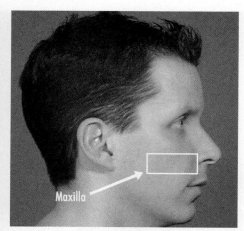

The maxilla is the bone that holds the upper row of teeth.

Palpation Example

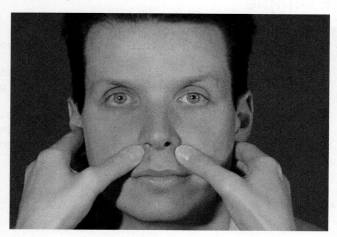

To palpate the maxilla,
1) Place the patient in a seated position at the end of the treatment table.
2) Using your fingertips or thumbs, locate the bone just above the upper row of teeth.
3) Palpate the bone starting at the midline of the face just below the nose, then move laterally, staying superior to the teeth and gums.

Nasal Bone

Skeletal and Anatomical Landmarks

Skeletal   **Anatomical**

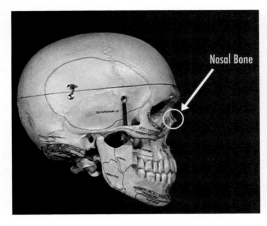
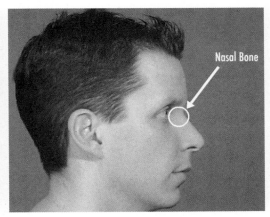

The nasal bone is located in the proximal half of the nose.

Palpation Example

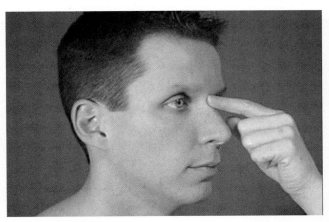

To palpate the nasal bone,
1) Place the patient in a seated position at the end of the treatment table.
2) The nasal bone is located in the proximal half of the nose. Using your thumb, index, and middle fingers, gently grasp the nose, palpating the bone from the nose's junction with the forehead to the midpoint of the nose.
3) You may need to stabilize the back of the patient's head with your other hand.

◉ Orbit

Skeletal and Anatomical Landmarks

Skeletal   **Anatomical**

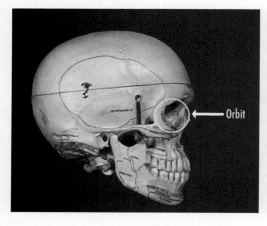   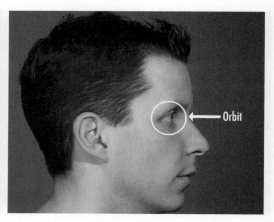

The orbit of the eye is the eye socket.

Palpation Example

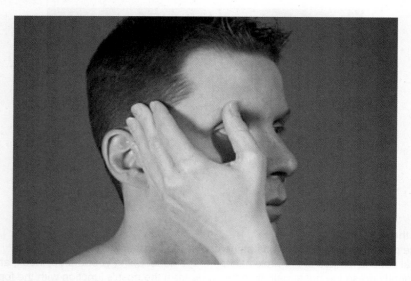

To palpate the orbit of the eye,
1) Place the patient in a seated position at the end of the treatment table.
2) Stabilize the patient's head with one hand, and palpate with the other hand.
3) If needed, stabilize the palpating hand by gently touching your fingers against the patient's face.
4) Use your thumb to gently palpate the bony ridge that surrounds the entire eye.

Scalene Muscles

Skeletal and Anatomical Landmarks

Skeletal

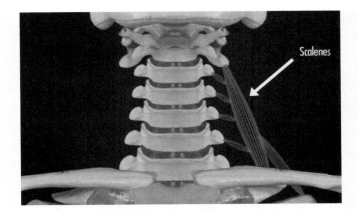

Anatomical

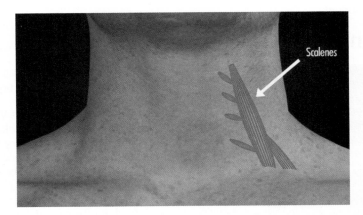

The scalene muscles lie deep in the lateral neck, posterior to the sternocleidomastoid muscle and anterior to the upper trapezius.

Palpation Example

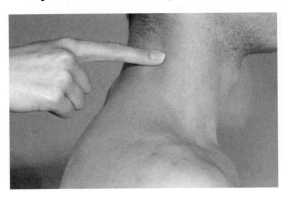

To palpate the scalenes,
1) Place the patient in a seated position at the end of the treatment table.
2) Using 2–3 fingers, press in the lateral neck region, posterior to the sternocleido-mastoid muscle and anterior to the upper trapezius muscle.
3) The scalenes lie deeper in this triangular area.

◉ Sternal (Jugular) Notch

Skeletal and Anatomical Landmarks

Skeletal   **Anatomical**

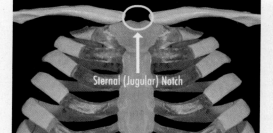   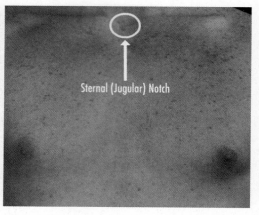

The sternal notch (also called the jugular notch) is the V-shaped divot located on the superior aspect of the manubrium.

Palpation Example

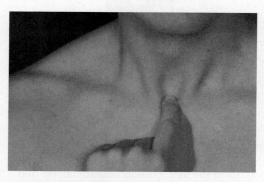

To palpate the sternal (also called jugular) notch,
1) Place the patient in a seated position at the end of the treatment table.
2) Place your finger gently in the V-shaped divot at the anterior base of the neck, then
3) Press inferiorly to feel the bony notch.
4) To make the sternal notch become more prominent, ask the patient to flex the neck (against resistance, if necessary).
5) The sternocleidomastoid muscles outline the borders of the sternal notch area.

TIP

Flex Neck

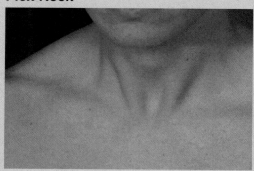

To make the sternal notch become more prominent, ask the patient to flex the neck (against resistance, if necessary).

⦿ Sternocleidomastoid Muscle

Skeletal and Anatomical Landmarks

Skeletal   **Anatomical**

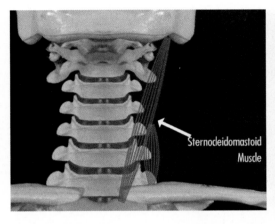 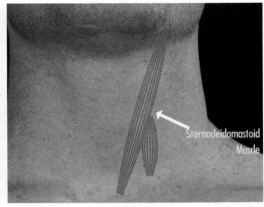

The sternocleidomastoid muscle has two heads that originate on the medial clavicle and the manubrium. The heads joint together to insert on the mastoid process.

Palpation Example

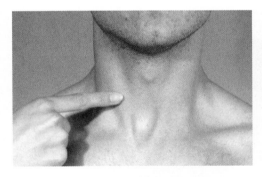 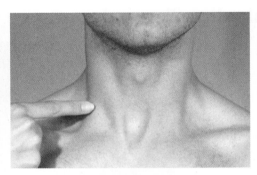

To palpate the sternocleidomastoid muscle,
1) Place the patient in a seated position at the end of the treatment table.
2) Ask the patient to flex the neck and slightly rotate the head to the opposite side.
3) Gentle resistance will make the muscle become more identifiable.
4) Using your fingers, palpate the muscle that becomes very prominent on the anterior lateral neck from the mastoid process to the clavicle and manubrium.

◉ Temporomandibular Joint

Skeletal and Anatomical Landmarks

Skeletal   **Anatomical**

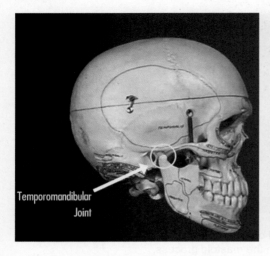
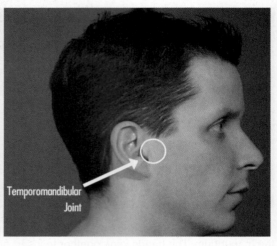

The temporomandibular joint is located just anterior to the tragus of the ear. It is the joint between the condylar process of the mandible and the temporal bone.

Palpation Example

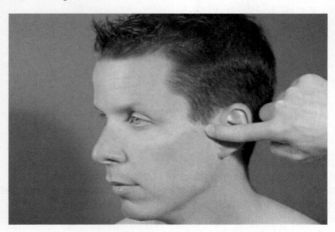

To palpate the temporomandibular joint,
1) Place the patient in a seated position at the end of the treatment table.
2) Locate the tragus of the ear, then
3) Move anteriorly about one finger width to a bony knob.
4) The bony knob is the condylar process of the mandible.
5) Ask the patient to open and close the jaw.
6) When the jaw opens, you will feel the condylar process move anteriorly and inferiorly, opening the temporomandibular joint and leaving a small divot in the joint socket.

Alternate View

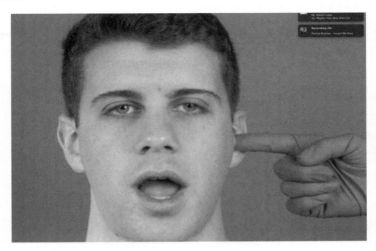

Alternate Method:
1) Using a gloved hand, gently place the index finger in the ear with pressure against the anterior portion of the ear near the tragus.
2) Ask the patient to open and close the jaw.
3) The joint will be felt as the jaw moves.

TIP

Open and Close the Jaw

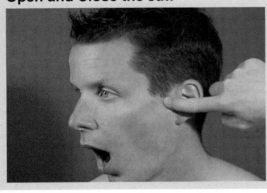

With the fingers over the temporomandibular joint, ask the patient to open and close the jaw. You will feel the joint open and a larger divot appear, verifying a correct palpation.

◉ Thyroid Cartilage

Skeletal and Anatomical Landmarks

Skeletal

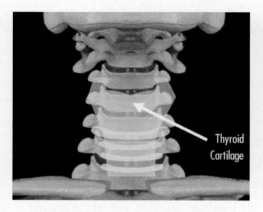

Thyroid
Cartilage

Anatomical

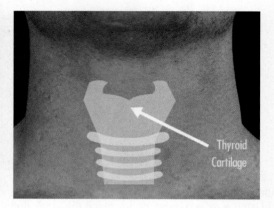

Thyroid
Cartilage

The thyroid cartilage is located in the anterior neck region. The upper portion of the thyroid cartilage is easily palpated due to its prominent notch known commonly as the Adam's Apple.

Palpation Example

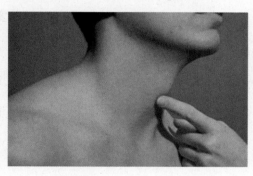

To palpate the thyroid cartilage,
1) Place the patient in a seated position at the end of the treatment table.
2) Run your finger gently down the anterior aspect of the throat until a notch is felt, then
3) Proceed further to the large protrusion.
   This protrusion is the upper notch/lip of the thyroid cartilage and is often referred to as the "Adam's Apple."
4) The lower portion of the thyroid cartilage is located just beneath the lip and extends approximately 1–2 finger widths inferiorly.

TIP
Swallow

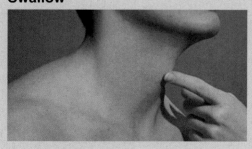

To better visualize the thyroid cartilage, ask the patient to swallow. The thyroid cartilage will move up and down with the swallowing maneuver.

● Zygomatic Arch

Skeletal and Anatomical Landmarks

Skeletal   **Anatomical**

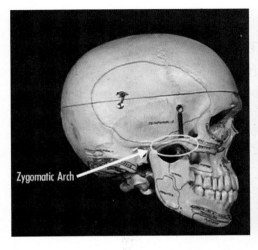
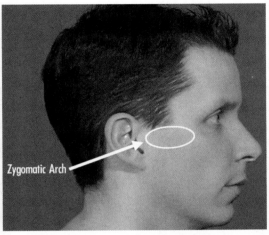

The zygomatic arch is often referred to as the cheek bone. It is the ridge of bone that starts below the orbit and extends toward the ear.

Palpation Example

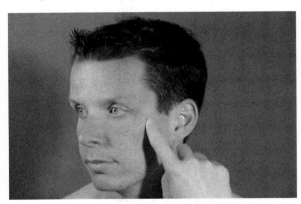

To palpate the zygomatic arch,
1) Place the patient in a seated position at the end of the treatment table.
2) Using your fingers, locate the longer ridgelike bone that lies between the sharper cheek bone and the ear.
3) The zygomatic arch can be palpated from the hairline (superior and anterior to the temporomandibular joint) to the zygomatic bone (cheek bone) that is just lateral and inferior to the eye socket.

● Manubrium

Skeletal and Anatomical Landmarks

Skeletal

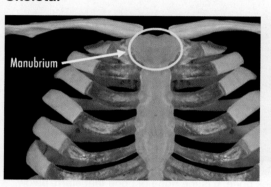

Anatomical

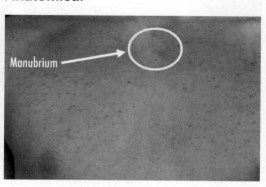

The manubrium is the superior-most aspect of the sternum.

Palpation Example

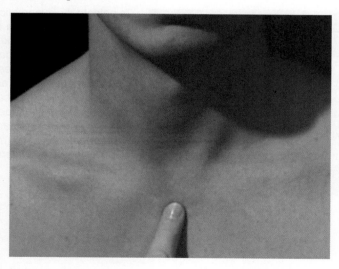

To palpate the manubrium,
1) Place the patient in a seated position at the end of the treatment table.
2) Locate the sternal notch. This is the superior-most portion of the manubrium.
3) Move your finger inferiorly onto the flat portion of the bone.
4) The manubrium is the superior portion of the sternum and can be palpated from the sternal notch inferiorly 2–3 finger widths.

● Sternum

Skeletal and Anatomical Landmarks

Skeletal

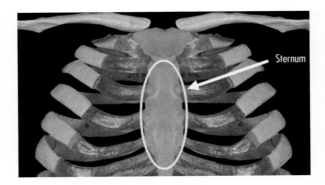

Anatomical

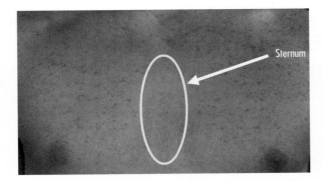

The sternum is the bone often referred to as the breast bone.

Palpation Example

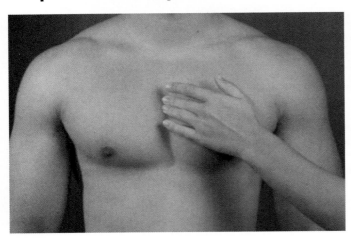

To palpate the sternum,
1) Place the patient in a seated position at the end of the treatment table.
2) Locate the bone just inferior to the manubrium.
3) Palpate the sternum (the bone that is commonly referred to as the breast bone) from the manubrium to the inferior notch where the xiphoid process is located.

◉ Xiphoid Process

Skeletal and Anatomical Landmarks

Skeletal   **Anatomical**

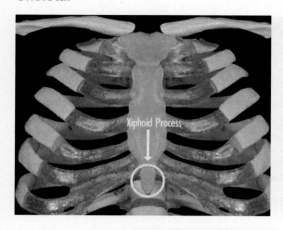   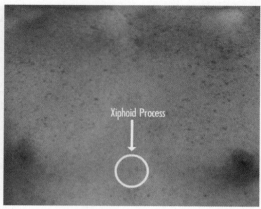

The xiphoid process is the small, pointed cartilage structure at the distal end of the sternum.

Palpation Example

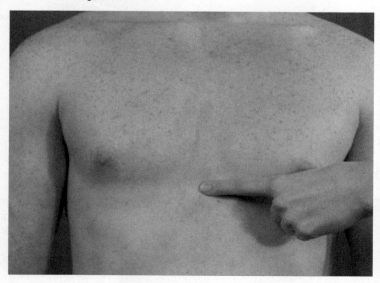

To palpate the xiphoid process,
1) Place the patient in a seated position at the end of the treatment table or standing.
2) Locate the xiphoid process by following the ribs proximally to the notch where the left and right sides join.
3) The xiphoid process lies in this small notch or "divot" and extends approximately two finger widths distally from this point.

● Acromioclavicular Joint

Skeletal and Anatomical Landmarks

Skeletal   **Anatomical**

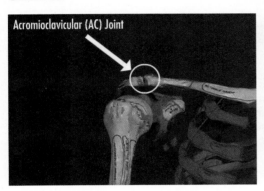

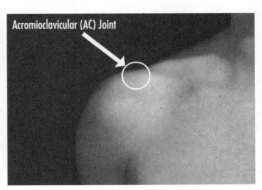

The acromioclavicular joint (AC joint) is located on the superior aspect of the shoulder and is the articulation of the clavicle and the acromion process.

Palpation Example

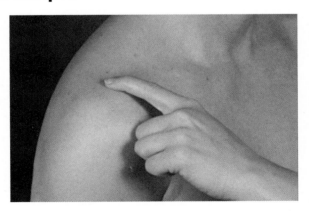

To palpate the AC joint,
1) Place the patient in a seated position at the end of the treatment table. Stand in front or to the side of the patient.
2) Locate the clavicle and follow it to the lateral end.
3) The end of the clavicle is distinguished from the shaft by a larger bony bump on the top of the shoulder.
4) Proceed a few millimeters beyond that bump laterally until you feel a slight drop-off or groove. This groove is the AC joint.
5) Moving your finger anteriorly and posteriorly along the groove will allow you to palpate the AC ligament that crosses the joint.

TIP

#1: Abduct the Shoulder

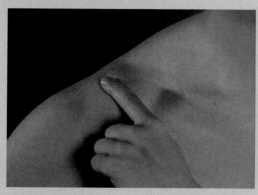

To verify that you are on the AC joint, hold your finger on the joint and ask the patient to abduct and adduct the arm. You should feel movement of the joint under your finger.

#2: Abduct and Depress the Shoulder

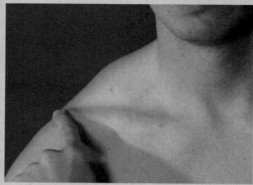

To verify that you are on the AC joint, hold your finger on the joint and ask the patient to simultaneously depress the shoulder and abduct the arm. You should feel movement of the joint under your finger.

● Acromion Process

Skeletal and Anatomical Landmarks

Skeletal

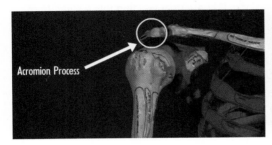

Anatomical

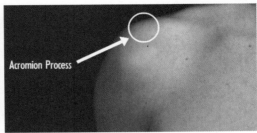

The acromion process is the extension of the scapular spine and lies lateral to the end of the clavicle at the "tip" of the shoulder.

Palpation Example

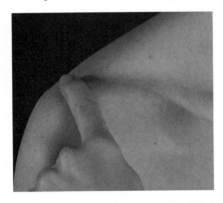

To palpate the acromion process,
1) Place the patient in a seated position at the end of the treatment table. Stand in front or to the side of the patient.
2) Grasp the superior-anterior and posterior shoulder between the thumb and fingers.
3) Locate the sharper bony protrusion on the lateral posterior edge of the superior shoulder. That bony prominence is the posterior lateral portion of the acromion process.
4) From that location, trace the bony ridge along the lateral border, then roll the finger up on top of the large flat bone. That flat bone is the superior aspect of the acromion process.

TIP

#1: Lateral Edge

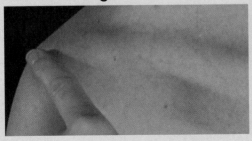

You can confirm your palpation of the acromion process by feeling for the distinct bony drop-off on the superior lateral edge of the shoulder. Locate that edge, then move back up on top of the plateau. That plateau is the acromion process.

#2: Divot

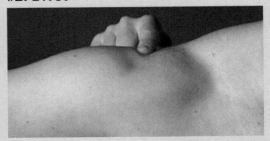

With the arm abducted, place your finger in the divot created medial to the deltoid muscles on the top of the shoulder. This location should be the acromion process. Hold your finger in place and ask the patient to lower the arm, then verify that you are on the acromion process by feeling for its sharp lateral edge.

TIP

#3: Posterior Edge

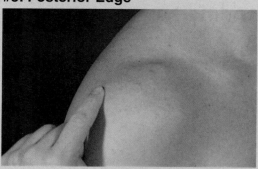

The posterior lateral edge of the acromion is the most prominent aspect of the bone and can help you locate the rest of the bone. Palpate until you find this distinct bony protrusion at the posterior lateral corner of the shoulder, then follow the ridge anteriorly along the shoulder. Once at the midpoint of the shoulder, slide your finger up on top of the plateau. You will be at the center of the acromion process.

Anterior Deltoid Muscle

Skeletal and Anatomical Landmarks

Skeletal

Anatomical

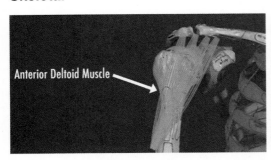

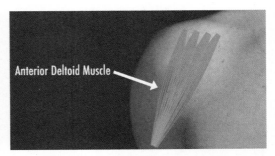

The anterior deltoid muscle is the front one-third of the larger muscle mass on the proximal humerus. It originates on the clavicle and inserts at the deltoid tubercle.

Palpation Example

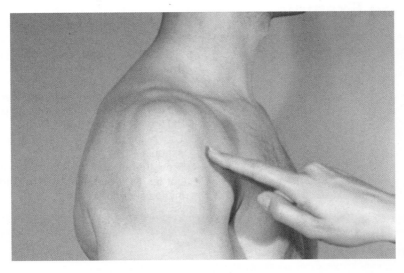

To palpate the anterior deltoid muscle,
1) Place the patient in a seated position at the end of the treatment table. Stand in front or to the side of the patient.
2) Ask the patient to gently flex the shoulder against resistance, exposing the anterior portion of the muscle that "caps" the shoulder.
3) Locate the portion of the muscle that originates from the lateral clavicle and follow it inferiorly and laterally along the anterior humerus about 4 to 6 inches to its insertion at the deltoid tubercle.
4) The muscle can be palpated with a single digit or by gently pinching it between the thumb and fingers.

◉ Axillary Border of the Scapula

Skeletal and Anatomical Landmarks

Skeletal

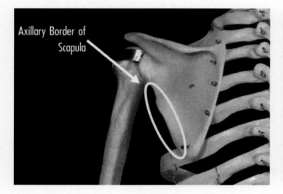

Anatomical

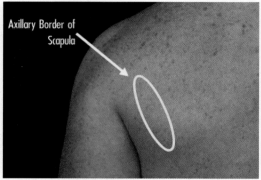

The axillary border of the scapula refers to the lateral border.

Palpation Example

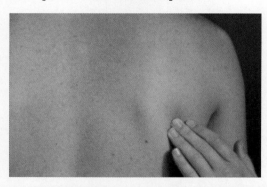

To palpate the axillary border of the scapula,
1) Place the patient in a seated position at the end of the treatment table. Stand to the side of the patient.
2) If the patient is able, ask the patient to bring his or her hand of the side being palpated behind his or her back.
3) Locate the prominent inferior angle of the scapula.
4) From there, follow the bony ridge of the lateral border of the scapula (axillary border) several inches superiorly.

TIP

Arm Behind Back

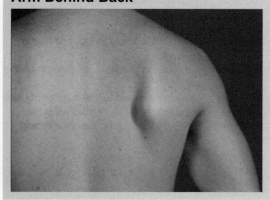

To allow the scapula to become more prominent, ask the patient to place his or her forearm on his or her low back.

⊙ Bicipital Groove

Skeletal and Anatomical Landmarks

Skeletal

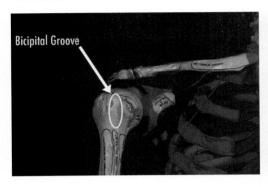

Anatomical

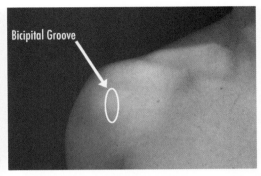

The bicipital groove lies between the greater and lesser tubercles of the humerus.

Palpation Example

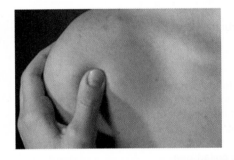

To palpate the bicipital groove,
1) Place the patient in a seated position at the end of the treatment table. Stand facing the patient.
2) With the patient's forearm resting on his or her thigh, locate the greater tubercle.
3) From the greater tubercle, move one finger width medially and slightly inferiorly.
4) The bicipital groove should be under your finger and can be felt for a length of approximately ½ to 1 inch.

TIP

Three Landmarks

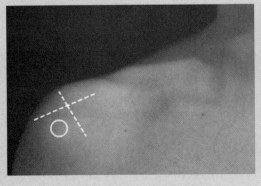

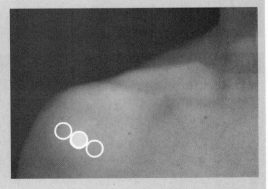

1) The bicipital groove is the second landmark in a row of three landmarks.
2) Once the greater tubercle is located, place three fingers next to each other in a descending, medially slanting pattern.
3) From lateral to medial, the fingers should be on the greater tubercle, the bicipital groove, and the lesser tubercle.

◉ Clavicle

Skeletal and Anatomical Landmarks

Skeletal   **Anatomical**

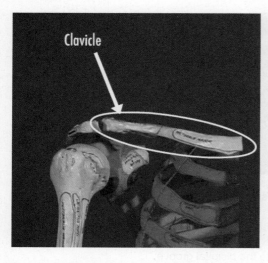

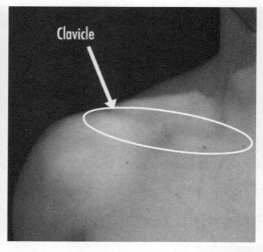

The clavicle is the bone commonly referred to as the collarbone.

Palpation Example

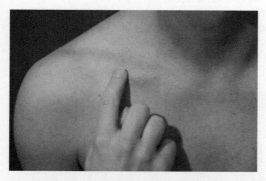

To palpate the clavicle,
1) Place the patient in a seated position at the end of the treatment table. Stand in front of the patient.
2) Locate the long, narrow bone often referred to as the collarbone.
3) Palpate along its full length from the sternoclavicular joint to the AC joint with the flats of one or two fingers.

TIP

#1: Round Shoulders

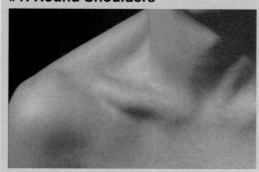

The clavicle is more prominent if the patient rounds the shoulders forward, cupping the chest.

◉ Coracoid Process

Skeletal and Anatomical Landmarks

Skeletal   **Anatomical**

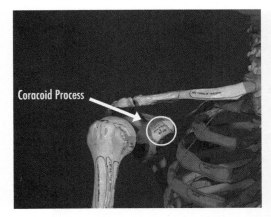

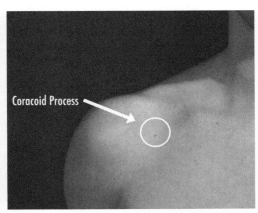

The coracoid process is located inferior to the clavicle and medial to the lesser tubercle of the humerus.

Palpation Example

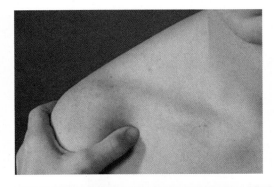

To palpate the coracoid process,
1) Place the patient in a seated position at the end of the treatment table. Stand slightly to the side of the patient.
2) Locate the coracoid process by placing the heel of your hand on the anterior shoulder/ chest area inferior to the distal clavicle and medial to the shoulder.
3) Feel for a large fingerlike, bony protrusion, which is the coracoid process.
4) Once located, palpate the coracoid process with one finger or the thumb.

TIP

Heel of Hand

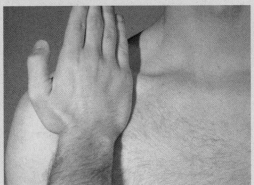

To initially locate the coracoid process, the evaluator may place the heel on the anterior shoulder/chest area to feel for the bony protrusion of the coracoid.

◉ Deltoid Tubercle

Skeletal and Anatomical Landmarks

Skeletal   **Anatomical**

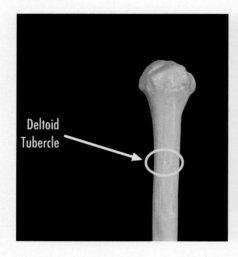

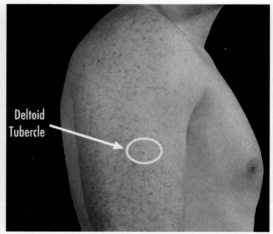

The deltoid tubercle is located approximately one-third of the way down the lateral aspect of the humerus and serves as the attachment site for the deltoid muscles.

Palpation Example

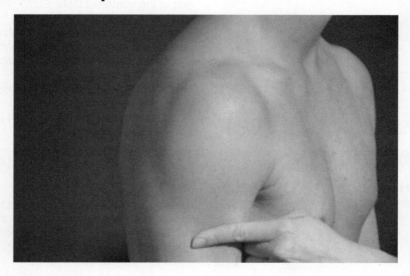

To palpate the deltoid tubercle,
1) Place the patient in a seated position at the end of the treatment table. Stand in front or to the side of the patient.
2) Place the flat of your finger on the mid deltoid muscle then move your finger inferiorly along the deltoid while applying gentle inward pressure.
3) You will feel an indentation or groove at the inferior edge of the deltoid muscle, about one-third to one-half the way down the humerus.
4) The deltoid tubercle lies at the center of this groove.

● Greater Tubercle

Skeletal and Anatomical Landmarks

Skeletal   **Anatomical**

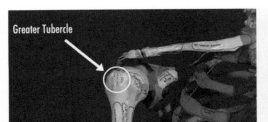

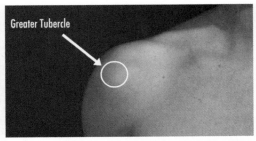

The greater tubercle lies on the superior aspect of the humerus just off the anterior lateral edge of the acromion process at approximately 45 degrees between the frontal and sagittal planes.

Palpation Example

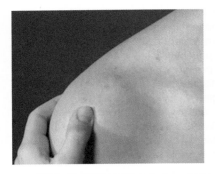

To palpate the greater tubercle,
1) Place the patient in a seated position at the end of the treatment table.
2) First locate the anterior lateral edge of the acromion process.
3) Move about one finger width off the acromion at a 45-degree angle between the frontal and sagittal planes.
4) The greater tubercle will be felt as a larger bony protrusion.
5) To verify that you are on the greater tubercle, ask the patient to internally and externally rotate the arm. You will feel the tubercle roll back and forth under your finger.

TIP

Verifying Landmark   **Row of Landmarks**

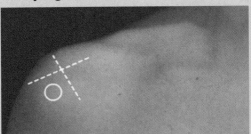

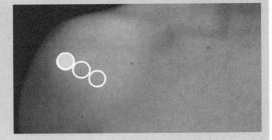

1) The greater tubercle is the first landmark in a row of three landmarks.
2) Once the greater tubercle is located, place three fingers next to each other in a descending, medially slanting pattern.
3) From lateral to medial, the fingers should be on the greater tubercle, the bicipital groove, and the lesser tubercle.

◉ Inferior Angle of Scapula

Skeletal and Anatomical Landmarks

Skeletal

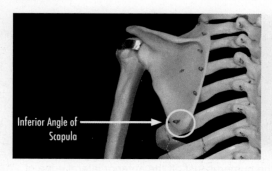

Inferior Angle of Scapula →

Anatomical

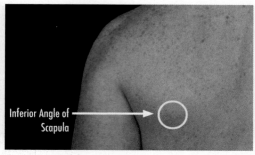

Inferior Angle of Scapula →

The inferior angle of the scapula is the prominent distal portion of the scapula.

Palpation Example

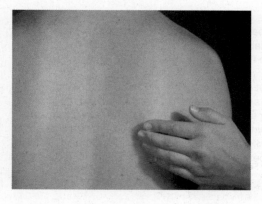

To palpate the inferior angle of the scapula,
1) Place the patient in a seated position at the end of the treatment table. Stand to the side or behind the patient.
2) Locate the prominent, most distal aspect of the scapula. This sharper curve in the bone is the inferior angle.
3) To easily locate the inferior angle of the scapula, ask the patient to place his or her forearm on his or her low back. This motion makes the inferior angle of the scapula protrude significantly.

TIP

Arm Behind Back

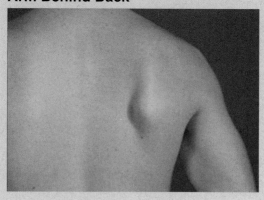

To allow the scapula to become more prominent, ask the patient to place his or her forearm on his or her low back.

● Infraspinatus Muscle

Skeletal and Anatomical Landmarks

Skeletal

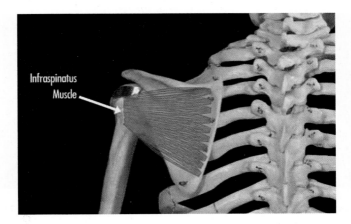

Anatomical

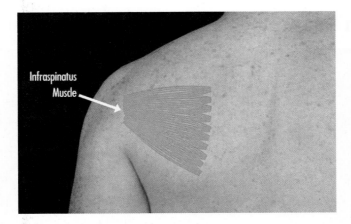

The infraspinatus muscle lies in the infraspinous fossa of the scapula and inserts on the greater tubercle. It is an external rotator of the shoulder.

Palpation Example

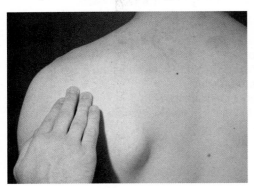

To palpate the infraspinatus muscle,
1) Place the patient in a seated position at the end of the treatment table. Stand to the side or behind the patient.
2) Locate the scapular spine.
3) Move inferiorly to the infraspinous fossa.
4) The muscle covers a majority of the fossa.
5) Palpate the entire infraspinous fossa area.

◉ Latissimus Dorsi Muscle

Skeletal and Anatomical Landmarks

Skeletal   **Anatomical**

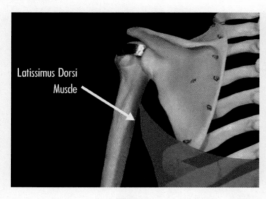
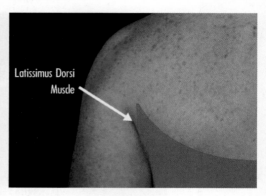

The latissimus dorsi muscles are the large flaring muscles located on the sides of the torso. They originate from lower thoracic and lumbar vertebrae and insert into the intertubercular groove of the humerus.

Palpation Example

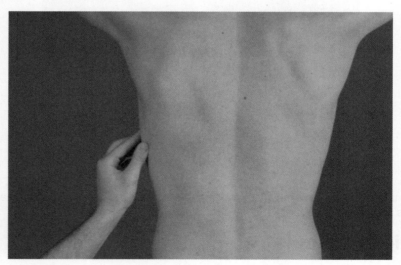

To palpate the latissimus dorsi muscle,
1) Place the patient either in a seated position at the end of the treatment table or standing.
2) Locate the large flaring muscles on the lateral torso.
3) Abducting the patient's arms to 90 degrees then applying slight resistance as the patient tries to adduct the arms will make the muscles become more prominent.
4) Palpate the full length of the muscle from the humerus to the torso.
5) The lateral portions of the muscle can be palpated by gently grasping the muscle between the thumb and fingers.

● Lesser Tubercle

Skeletal and Anatomical Landmarks

Skeletal **Anatomical**

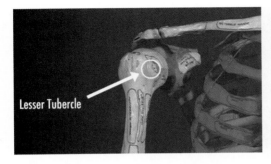 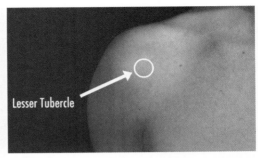

The lesser tubercle is the small bony protrusion on the superior humerus, medial to the bicipital groove. It serves as the attachment site for the subscapularis muscle.

Palpation Example

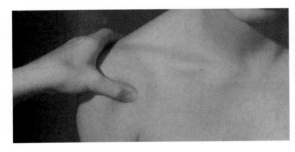

To palpate the lesser tubercle,
1) Place the patient in a seated position at the end of the treatment table.
2) Locate the greater tubercle.
3) Move two finger widths medially and slightly inferiorly.
4) The lesser tubercle is felt as a small bony protrusion and is more distinguishable when the humerus is rotated back and forth.

TIP

Three Landmarks in a Row

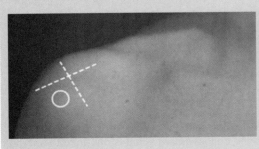 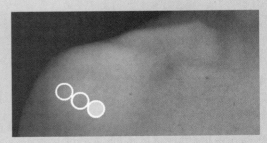

1) The lesser tubercle is the third landmark in a row of three landmarks.
2) Once the greater tubercle is located, place three fingers next to each other in a descending, medially slanting pattern.
3) From lateral to medial, the fingers should be on the greater tubercle, the bicipital groove, and the lesser tubercle.

◉ Mid Deltoid Muscle

Skeletal and Anatomical Landmarks

Skeletal   **Anatomical**

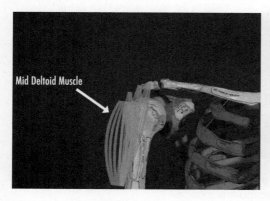
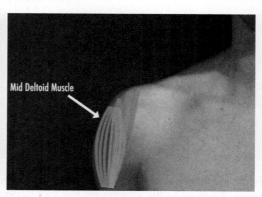

The mid deltoid muscle is the center, lateral-most portion of the deltoids.

Palpation Example

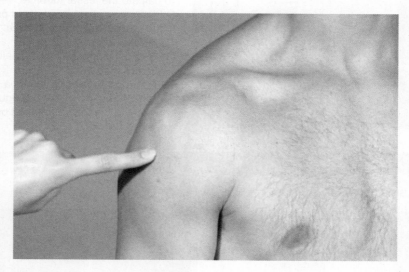

To palpate the mid deltoid muscle,
1) Place the patient in a seated position at the end of the treatment table.
2) Locate the acromion process.
3) Move laterally off the acromion onto the middle deltoid muscle.
4) Palpate the muscle from the acromion process to the deltoid tubercle that is one-third to one-half the way down the upper arm.

◉ Pectoralis Major Muscle

Skeletal and Anatomical Landmarks

Skeletal   **Anatomical**

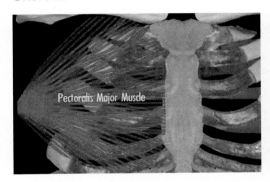
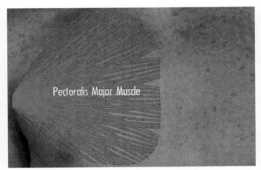

The pectoralis major muscle is the large fan-shaped muscle on the anterior chest. It has two heads, the sternal head and the clavicular head. The muscle arises from the medial clavicle, the sternum, and the costal cartilages of ribs 2 to 6 and inserts on the lateral lip of the bicipital groove.

Palpation Example

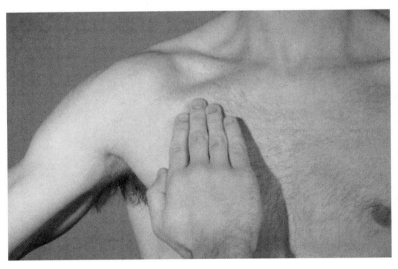

To palpate the pectoralis major muscle,
1) Place the patient in a seated position at the end of the treatment table or standing.
2) Locate the large anterior chest muscle.
3) Palpate its borders along the clavicle and sternum as well as the full surface of the muscle to its attachment on the upper humerus.

Posterior Deltoid Muscle

Skeletal and Anatomical Landmarks

Skeletal   **Anatomical**

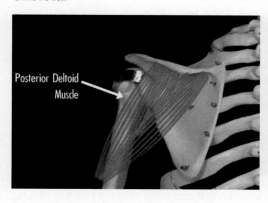
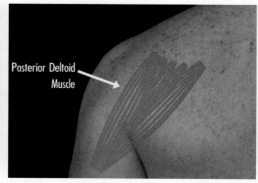

The posterior deltoid muscle is the back one-third of the deltoid. It originates on the scapular spine and inserts on the deltoid tubercle.

Palpation Example

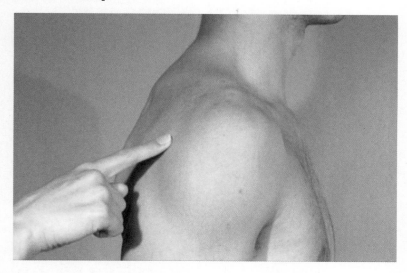

To palpate the posterior deltoid muscle,
1) Place the patient in a seated position at the end of the treatment table. Stand to the side of the patient.
2) The posterior deltoid muscle can be palpated by locating the posterior portion of the large muscle that caps the shoulder.
3) It can be palpated from the scapular spine to the deltoid tubercle.

● Spine of Scapula

Skeletal and Anatomical Landmarks

Skeletal   **Anatomical**

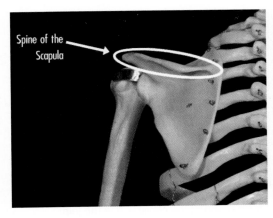
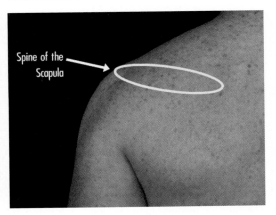

The spine of the scapula is the long, bony, horizontal ridge on the posterior-superior aspect of the scapula.

Palpation Example

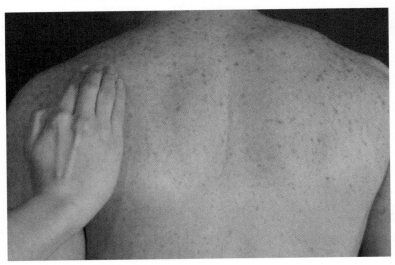

To palpate the spine of the scapula,
1) Place the patient in a seated position at the end of the treatment table. Stand to the side of the patient.
2) Starting with three or four fingers on the middle of the upper trapezius muscle region, draw your hand inferiorly down the scapula.
3) The spine of the scapula will be felt as a bony ridge on the superior scapula.
4) Palpate the full length of the scapular spine from the vertebral border to the acromion process.

◉ Sternoclavicular Joint

Skeletal and Anatomical Landmarks

Skeletal   **Anatomical**

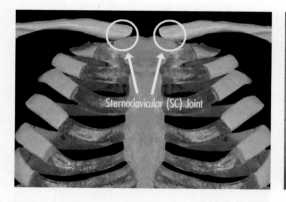
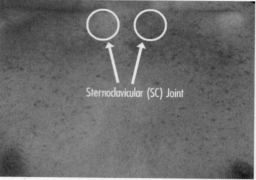

The sternoclavicular joint (SC joint) is located at the medial end of the clavicle. It is the joint between the sternum and the clavicle.

Palpation Example

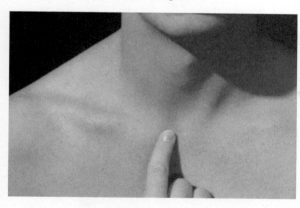

To palpate the SC joint,
1) Place the patient in a seated position at the end of the treatment table.
2) Locate the medial end of the clavicle which is felt like a ball-like protrusion.
3) The joint is just medial to this protrusion where the bone drops off.

TIPS

To verify the proper location of the SC joint,
1) Hold your finger on the joint and ask the patient to shrug the shoulders.
2) You should feel the movement of the joint under your finger.
3) To make the SC joint more prominent, ask the patient to round the shoulders then flex the neck slightly and turn the head to the opposite side.
4) This action makes the clavicle and sternocleidomastoid muscle become more prominent.
5) The SC joint is located at the junction of these two structures.

Subacromial Bursa

Skeletal and Anatomical Landmarks

Skeletal

Anatomical

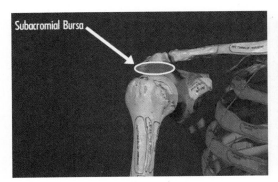
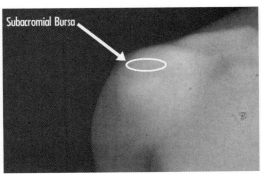

The subacromial bursa lies between the acromion process and head of the humerus.

Palpation Example

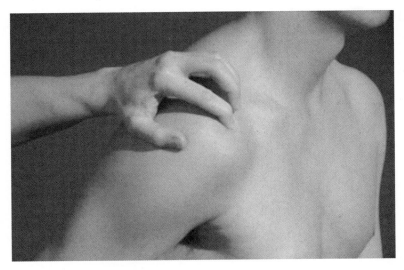

To palpate the subacromial bursa,
1) Place the patient in a seated position at the end of the treatment table.
2) Locate the anterior edge of the acromion process.
3) Move your finger forward until it drops onto the anterior aspect of the head of the humerus.
4) Holding your finger in place, ask the patient to extend the shoulder.
5) This motion causes the bursa to move from under the acromion to where it is palpable.
6) Unless the bursa is inflamed, it is difficult to distinguish.

◉ Superior Angle of Scapula

Skeletal and Anatomical Landmarks

Skeletal

Anatomical

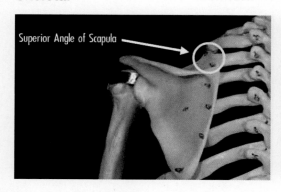 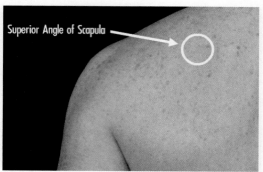

The superior angle of the scapula is the pointed portion of the bone superior to the scapular spine and anterior to the supraspinous fossa. It serves as the attachment site for the levator scapulae muscle.

Palpation Example

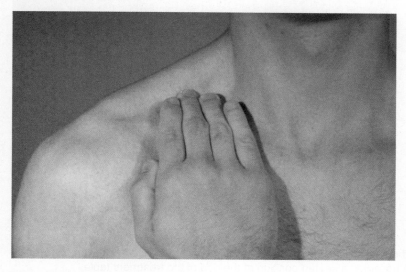

To palpate the superior angle of the scapula,
1) Place the patient in a seated position at the end of the treatment table.
2) Ask the patient to tilt the scapula anteriorly by placing the arm behind the back.
3) Using two or three fingers, palpate in the anterior triangular divot that is created between the clavicle and the upper trapezius muscle.
4) The superior angle of the scapula will be felt as a hard lump in the middle of the divot just inferior to the trapezius muscle.

Supraspinatus Muscle

Skeletal and Anatomical Landmarks

Skeletal

Anatomical

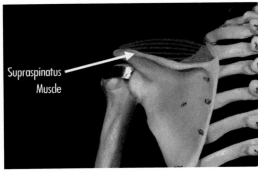

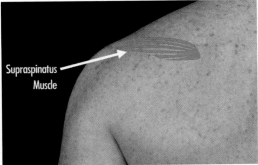

The supraspinatus muscle lies in the supraspinous fossa of the scapula and inserts on the greater tubercle of the humerus.

Palpation Example

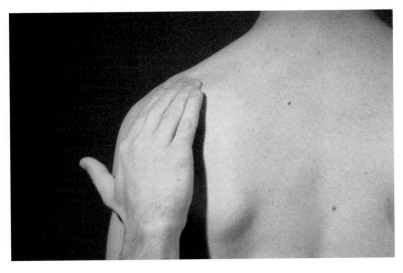

To palpate the supraspinatus muscle,
1) Place the patient in a seated position at the end of the treatment table.
2) Stand to the side of the patient.
3) Locate the spine of the scapula then move superiorly into the supraspinous fossa.
4) The supraspinatus muscle lies deep to the trapezius muscle in the fossa and should be palpated the full length of the supraspinous fossa.

● Teres Major Muscle

Skeletal and Anatomical Landmarks

Skeletal

Anatomical

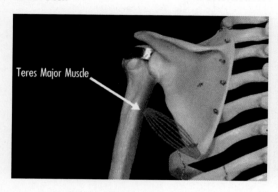

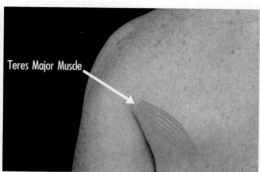

The teres major muscle arises from the inferior angle of the scapula and inserts on the medial lip of the bicipital groove.

Palpation Example

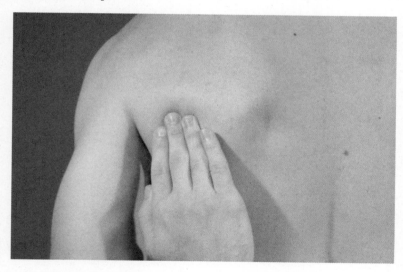

To palpate the teres major muscle,
1) Place the patient in a seated position at the end of the treatment table. Stand to the side of the patient.
2) Locate the infraspinatus muscle inferior to the spine of the scapula.
3) Move inferiorly and laterally to the lateral edge of the scapula.
4) The teres major muscle forms a fatter ridge as it extends in an upper sloping angle from the inferior angle of the scapula to the proximal humerus.

● Teres Minor Muscle

Skeletal and Anatomical Landmarks

Skeletal   **Anatomical**

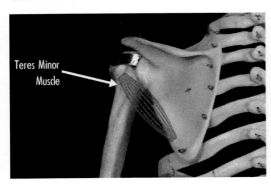
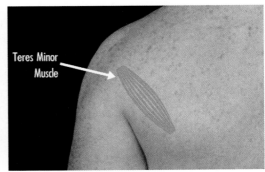

The teres minor muscle originates on the superior axillary border of the scapula and inserts on the greater tubercle of the humerus. It is an external rotator of the shoulder.

Palpation Example

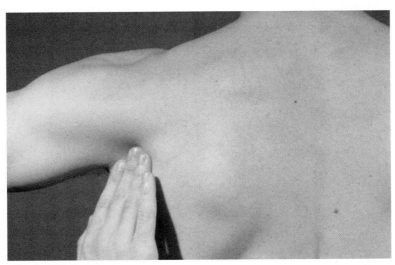

To palpate the teres minor muscle,
1) Place the patient in either a seated position at the end of the treatment table or standing. Stand to the side of the patient.
2) With the arm abducted to 90 degrees, visualize the teres major muscle and the divot that forms under the posterior deltoid muscle.
3) The teres minor muscle can be palpated just medial to the divot and superior to the teres major muscle.

◉ Trapezius Muscle (Upper)

Skeletal and Anatomical Landmarks

Skeletal   **Anatomical**

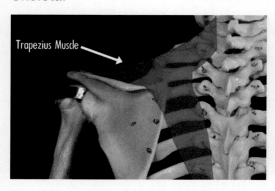
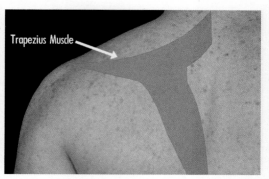

The trapezius muscle has three parts. Together, they extend from the occipital bone, ligamentum nuchae, and cervical and thoracic vertebrae to the posterior lateral clavicle, acromion process, and spine of the scapula.

Palpation Example

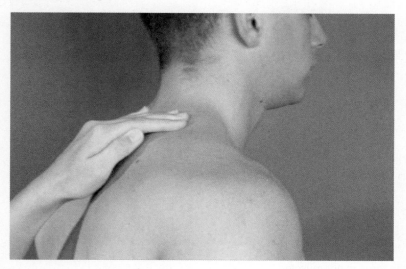

To palpate the upper trapezius muscle,
1) Place the patient in a seated position at the end of the treatment table.
2) Locate the larger flaring muscle on the superior shoulder. This muscle is the upper trapezius.
3) Palpate its length from the skull to the lateral clavicle. It can be palpated with the fingers or by gently pinching it between your fingers and thumb.

● Vertebral Border of the Scapula

Skeletal and Anatomical Landmarks

Skeletal

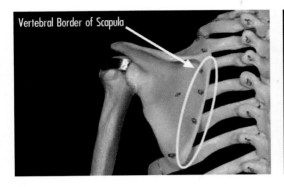

Anatomical

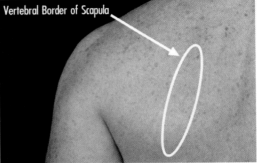

The vertebral border of the scapula is the side of the scapula closest to the spinal column. In a resting position, the vertebral border is vertical, parallel to the vertebrae.

Palpation Example

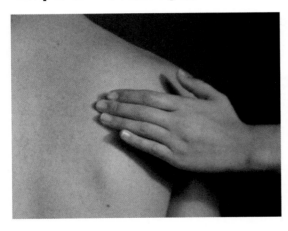

To palpate the vertebral border of the scapula,

1) Place the patient in a seated position at the end of the treatment table. Stand to the side of the patient.
2) If the patient is able, ask the patient to bring his or her hand of the side being palpated behind his or her back.
3) Locate the prominent inferior angle of the scapula.
4) From there, follow the bony ridge of the medial border of the scapula (vertebral border) several inches superiorly.

TIP

Arm Behind Back

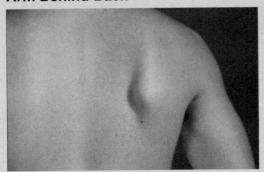

To allow the scapula to become more prominent, ask the patient to place his or her forearm on his or her low back.

● Annular Ligament

Skeletal and Anatomical Landmarks

Skeletal   **Anatomical**

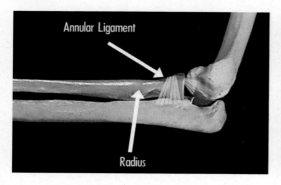

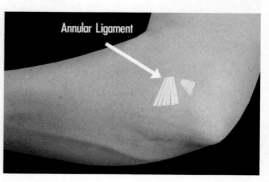

The annular ligament wraps around the head and neck of the radius, holding the radial head in place.

Palpation Example

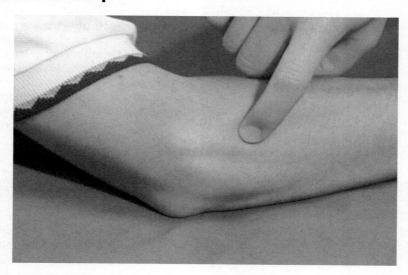

To palpate the annular ligament,
1) Place the patient's arm flexed at the elbow with their arm resting in front of their body.
2) Locate the radial head by moving 1–2 fingers widths distally from the lateral epicondyle.
3) Verify that you are on the radial head by supinating and pronating the forearm and feeling for the radial head to roll under your finger.
4) From there, move distally about ½ of a finger width. You will be on the neck of the radius.
5) The annular ligament will be under your finger, wrapping around the neck of the radius.

TIP

Four Landmarks

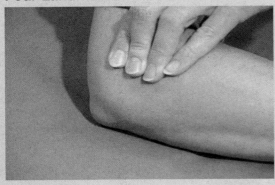

1) Locate the lateral epicondyle and hold one finger on the epicondyle.
2) Moving distally, place three more fingers down on the forearm along the radius.
3) The four fingers should be placed side-by-side touching each other.
4) The fingers will be located directly over four landmarks (proximal to distal): the lateral epicondyle, lateral collateral ligament, radial head, and annular ligament.

◉ Biceps Brachii Tendon

Skeletal and Anatomical Landmarks

Skeletal   **Anatomical**

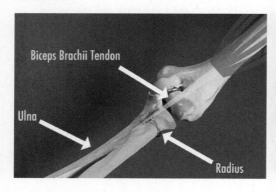

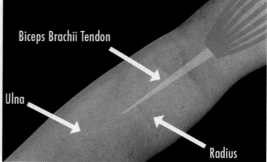

The distal biceps brachii tendon is located at the center of the anticubital fossa.

Palpation Example

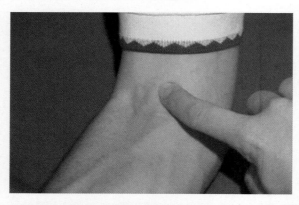

To palpate the bicep brachii tendon,
1) Place the patient in a seated position at the end of the treatment table or standing. Stand in front of the patient.
2) Ask the patient to flex the elbow and supinate the forearm.
3) Apply slight resistance if necessary.
4) Locate the most prominent tendon that lies near the center of the anterior crease of the elbow.
5) The tendon can be palpated with one digit or by gently pinching the tendon between the thumb and fingers.

TIP

Applying Resistance

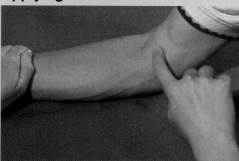

Applying resistance to the wrist as the patient flexes the elbow will cause the biceps brachii tendon to become more prominent.

⦿ Brachial Artery

Skeletal and Anatomical Landmarks

Skeletal

Anatomical

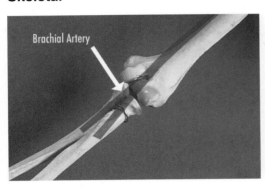
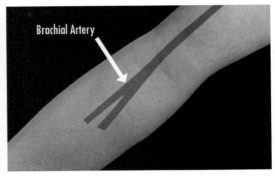

The brachial artery is located along the anterior medial humerus. It runs the length of the upper arm and through the cubital fossa.

Palpation Example

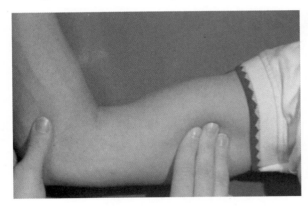

To palpate the brachial pulse/artery,
1) Place the patient in a seated position at the end of the treatment table.
2) Ask the patient to abduct and externally rotate the shoulder so the inner arm is exposed.
3) Using three fingers, press into the groove located at the midpoint of the inner upper arm, under the biceps muscle.
4) Use the flats of the distal phalanx to palpate the pulse.

Alternate Method

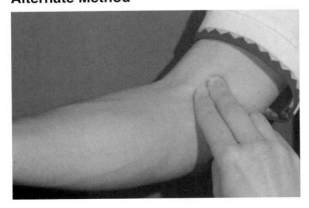

The brachial pulse can also be palpated at the cubital fossa. To palpate the artery, press your fingers gently into the cubital fossa just medial to the biceps tendon.

● Brachioradialis Muscle

Skeletal and Anatomical Landmarks

Skeletal

Anatomical

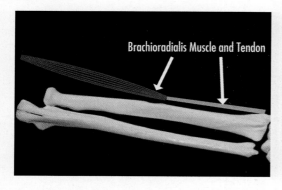

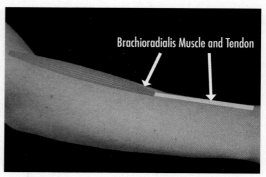

The brachioradialis muscle originates at the lateral supracondylar ridge of the humerus and inserts on the radius styloid.

Palpation Example

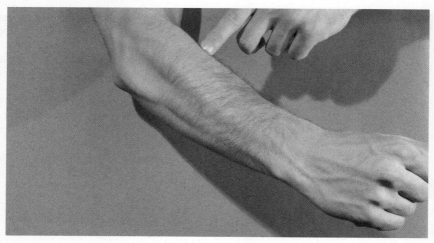

To palpate the brachioradialis muscle,
1) Place the patient in a seated position at the end of the treatment table.
2) Ask the patient to flex the elbow with the thumb pointing upward.
3) If possible, apply resistance.
4) The brachioradialis will become visible and palpable on the proximal forearm directly in line with the thumb.
5) The muscle can be palpated with the digits or by gently pinching the muscle between the thumb and fingers.
6) The muscle can be palpated from the elbow to its distal tendon.

● Common Extensor Tendon

Skeletal and Anatomical Landmarks

Skeletal   **Anatomical**

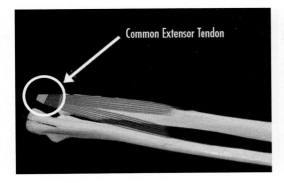

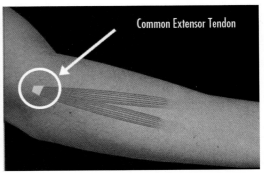

The common extensor tendon is the origin of the extensor muscles of the hand and wrist. It connects to the lateral epicondyle of the humerus.

Palpation Example

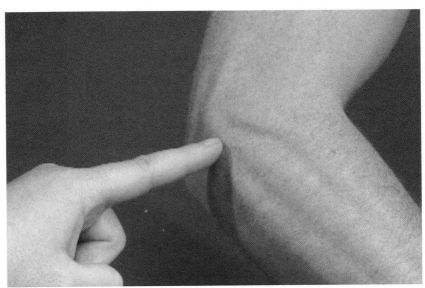

To palpate the common extensor tendon,
1) Place the patient in a seated position at the end of the treatment table with the elbow flexed.
2) Locate the lateral epicondyle of the humerus, then move distally just off the epicondyle and anterior to the radial collateral ligament.
3) The common extensor tendon can be felt as a larger band.
4) To verify you are on the tendon, ask the patient to gently extend the wrist.
5) The tendon will move under your finger.

● Common Flexor Tendon

Skeletal and Anatomical Landmarks

Skeletal

Anatomical

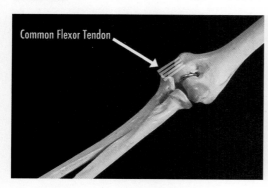

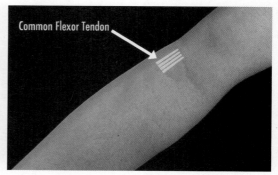

The common flexor tendon is the origin of the flexor muscles of the hand and wrist. It connects to the medial epicondyle of the humerus.

Palpation Example

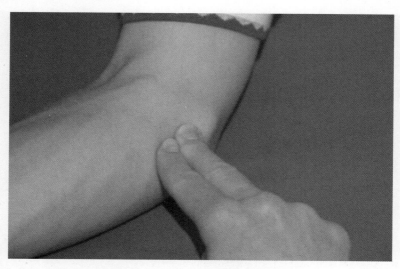

To palpate the common flexor tendon,
1) Place the patient in a seated position at the end of the treatment table with the elbow flexed and the forearm supinated.
2) Locate the medial epicondyle, then move distally and slightly anteriorly just off the epicondyle.
3) The tendon is felt as a thick band and can be palpated for 1–2 inches.
4) To verify you are on the tendon, ask the patient to gently flex the wrist. The tendon will move under your finger.

Cubital Fossa

Skeletal and Anatomical Landmarks

Skeletal

Anatomical

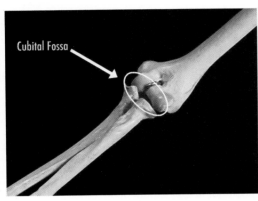

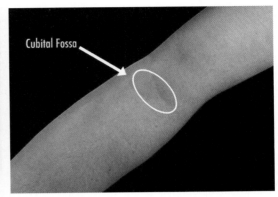

The cubital fossa is the depression region on the anterior crease of the elbow.

Palpation Example

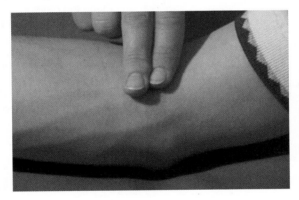

To palpate the cubital fossa,
1) Place the patient's forearm in a supinated position with the elbow slightly flexed.
2) The cubital fossa is the depression region on the anterior crease of the elbow.
3) Locate the depression and palpate its full width.

● Lateral Epicondyle of the Elbow

Skeletal and Anatomical Landmarks

Skeletal

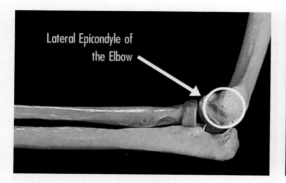

Lateral Epicondyle of
the Elbow

Anatomical

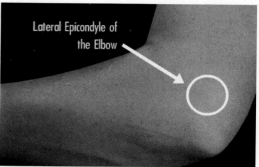

Lateral Epicondyle of
the Elbow

The lateral epicondyle of the elbow is located on the posterior lateral aspect of the elbow.

Palpation Example

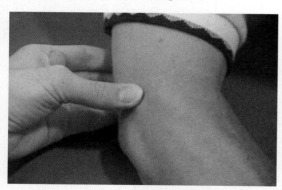

To palpate the lateral epicondyle of the elbow,
1) Place the patient's arm comfortably across the front of the body so the lateral aspect of the arm is visible.
2) Starting on the distal lateral humerus, move down the arm until the broadest part of the bone is felt.
3) The lateral epicondyle is the most prominent bone on the lateral elbow, just superior to the joint line.

TIP

Four Landmarks

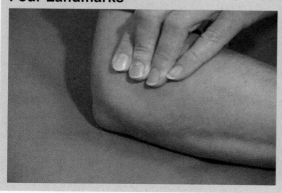

1) Locate the lateral epicondyle and hold one finger on the epicondyle.
2) Moving distally, place three more fingers down on the forearm along the radius. The four fingers should be placed side-by-side touching each other.
3) The fingers will be located directly over four landmarks (proximal to distal): the lateral epicondyle, lateral collateral ligament, radial head, and annular ligament.

● Lateral Supracondylar Ridge

Skeletal and Anatomical Landmarks

Skeletal   **Anatomical**

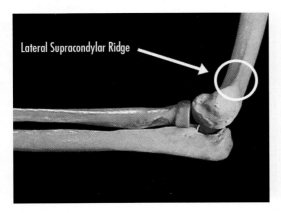
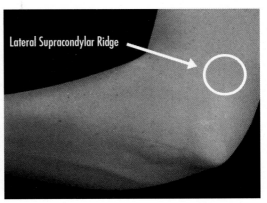

The lateral supracondylar ridge is the flared portion of the humerus just superior to the lateral epicondyle.

Palpation Example

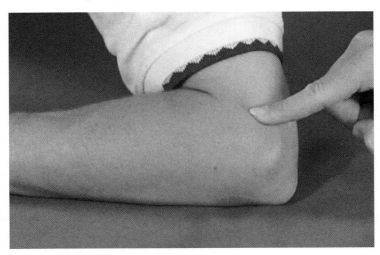

To palpate the lateral supracondylar ridge,
1) Place the patient's arm comfortably across the front of the body so the lateral aspect of the arm is visible.
2) Starting on the distal lateral humerus, move down the arm until you feel the bone "flare out" to the broadest part of the bone.
3) If you reach the lateral epicondyle, back up some to the "flared" part.
4) This flared part just superior to the epicondyle is the supracondylar ridge.

◉ Medial Epicondyle of the Elbow

Skeletal and Anatomical Landmarks

Skeletal   **Anatomical**

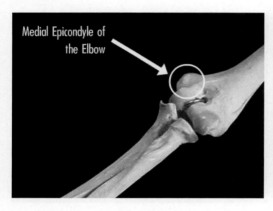   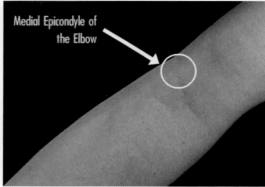

The medial epicondyle of the humerus is the large protruding bone on the inside of the elbow. It serves as the attachment site for the wrist flexors.

Palpation Example

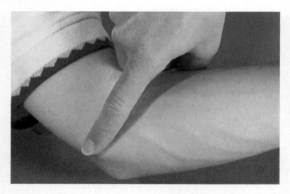

To palpate the medial epicondyle of the elbow,
1) Place the patient's arm in front of the body with the arm laterally rotated so the medial aspect of the arm is visible.
2) Starting on the distal medial humerus, move down the arm until the broadest part of the bone is felt.
3) The medial epicondyle is the most prominent bone on the medial elbow.

◉ Medial Supracondylar Ridge

Skeletal and Anatomical Landmarks

Skeletal

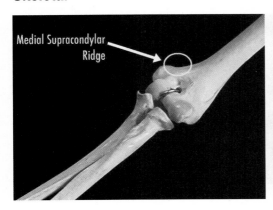

Medial Supracondylar
Ridge

Anatomical

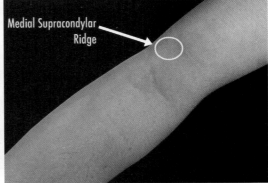

Medial Supracondylar
Ridge

The medial supracondylar ridge is the flared portion of the humerus just superior to the medial epicondyle.

Palpation Example

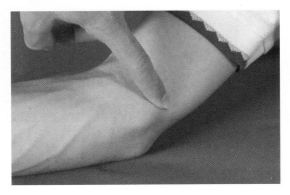

To palpate the medial supracondylar ridge,
1) Place the patient's arm in front of the body with the arm laterally rotated so the medial aspect of the arm is visible.
2) Starting on the distal medial humerus, move down the arm until you feel the bone "flare out" to the broadest part of the bone.
3) If you reach the medial epicondyle, back up some to the "flared" part.
4) This flared part just superior to the epicondyle is the supracondylar ridge.

⊙ Olecranon Bursa

Skeletal and Anatomical Landmarks

Skeletal

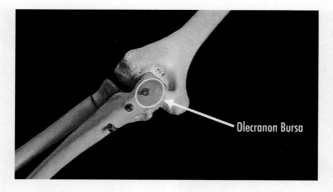

Olecranon Bursa

Anatomical

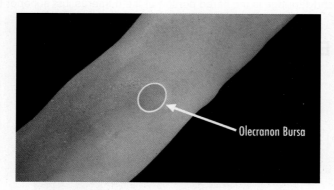

Olecranon Bursa

The olecranon bursa lies superficial to the olecranon process.

Palpation Example

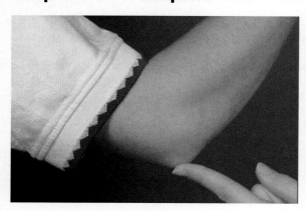

To palpate the olecranon bursa,
1) Place the patient in a seated position at the end of the treatment table with the elbow bent and the arm resting comfortably across the front of the body.
2) Because the olecranon bursa lies on the olecranon process, locate the olecranon process (bony peak of the elbow) and palpate the superficial surface of the process.
3) The olecranon bursa may not be detectable unless it is inflamed.

◉ Olecranon Fossa

Skeletal and Anatomical Landmarks

Skeletal

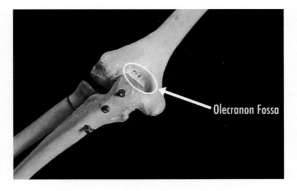

Anatomical

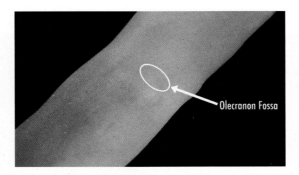

The olecranon fossa is the large divot in the posterior distal humerus that accepts the olecranon process when the elbow is extended.

Palpation Example

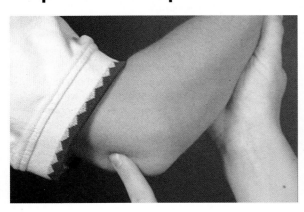

To palpate the olecranon fossa,
1) Place the patient in a seated position at the end of the treatment table with the elbow bent and the arm resting comfortably across the front of the body.
2) Locate the olecranon process which is the tip of the elbow, then
3) Move proximally about 1 inch until a large divot is felt on the distal humerus.
4) This divot is the olecranon fossa.

⦿ Olecranon Process

Skeletal and Anatomical Landmarks

Skeletal

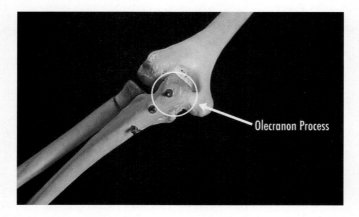

Olecranon Process

Anatomical

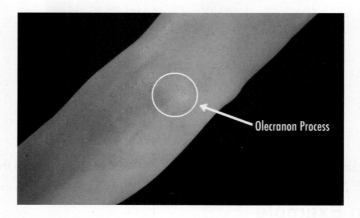

Olecranon Process

The olecranon process is the large bony protrusion at the tip of the elbow.

Palpation Example

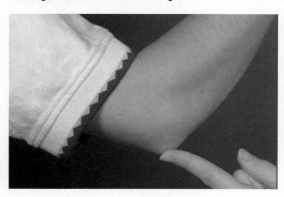

To palpate the olecranon process,
1) Place the patient in a seated position at the end of the treatment table with the elbow bent and the arm resting comfortably across the front of the body.
2) Locate the bony protrusion that forms the "peak" of the elbow.
3) This bone is the olecranon process.
4) Palpate the full surface of the bone.

● Radial (Lateral) Collateral Ligament

Skeletal and Anatomical Landmarks

Skeletal   **Anatomical**

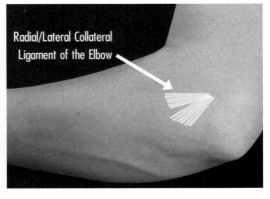

The radial collateral ligament of the elbow (lateral collateral ligament) is located between the lateral epicondyle and the radial head.

Palpation Example

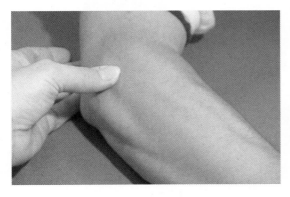

To palpate the radial (lateral) collateral ligament of the elbow,

1) Place the patient in a seated position at the end of the treatment table with the elbow bent and the arm resting comfortably across the front of the body so the lateral aspect of the arm is visible.
2) Locate the lateral epicondyle, then
3) Move distally toward the radial head.
4) The radial collateral ligament can be felt as a small band between the epicondyle and the radial head when anterior-posterior pressure is applied.

TIP

Four Landmarks

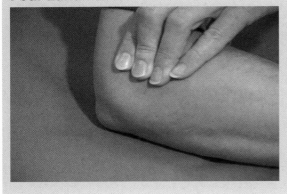

1) Locate the lateral epicondyle and hold one finger on the epicondyle.
2) Moving distally, place three more fingers down on the forearm along the radius.
3) The four fingers should be placed side-by-side touching each other.
4) The fingers will be located directly over four landmarks (proximal to distal): the lateral epicondyle, lateral collateral ligament, radial head, and annular ligament.

⦿ Radial Head

Skeletal and Anatomical Landmarks

Skeletal   **Anatomical**

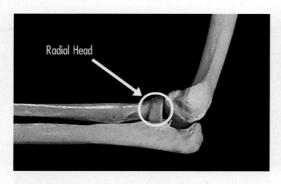

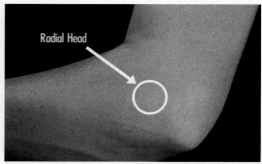

The radial head is located on the lateral forearm just distal to the lateral epicondyle of the humerus.

Palpation Example

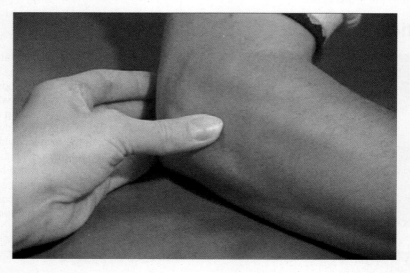

To palpate the radial head,
1) Position the patient with the elbow bent and the arm resting comfortably across the front of the body.
2) Locate the lateral epicondyle, then move distally approximately 1½–2 finger widths (or about 1 inch).
3) The radial head is felt as a bony knob on the posterio-lateral aspect of the elbow.
4) To confirm that you are palpating the radial head, ask the patient to supinate and pronate the forearm while your finger or thumb is on the bony prominence.
5) The radial head can be felt as a firm ball that rolls back and forth under your finger during these motions.

TIP

Confirming the Palpation

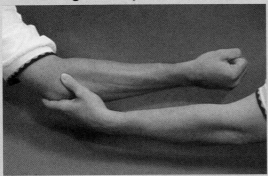

To confirm that you are palpating the radial head, ask the patient to supinate and pronate the forearm while your finger or thumb is on the bony prominence. If you are on the radial head, you will feel the bone roll back and forth under your finger during the supination and pronation movements.

Four Landmarks

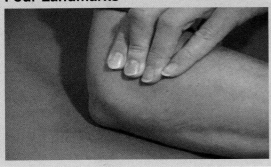

1) Locate the lateral epicondyle and hold one finger on the epicondyle.
2) Moving distally, place three more fingers down on the forearm along the radius. The four fingers should be placed side-by-side touching each other.
3) The fingers will be located directly over four landmarks (proximal to distal): the lateral epicondyle, lateral collateral ligament, radial head and annular ligament.

◉ Ulnar (Medial) Collateral Ligament

Skeletal and Anatomical Landmarks

Skeletal

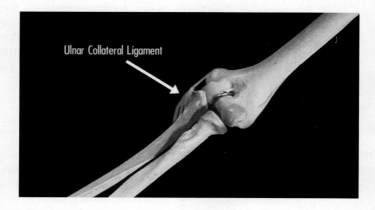

Ulnar Collateral Ligament

Anatomical

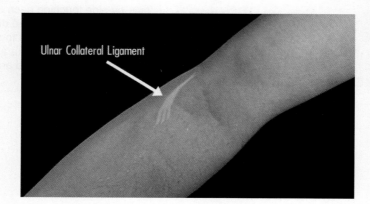

Ulnar Collateral Ligament

The ulnar collateral ligament attaches proximally to the medial epicondyle of the humerus and distally to the ulna.

Palpation Example

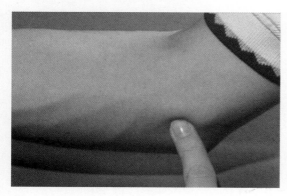

To palpate the ulnar (medial) collateral ligament,
1) Place the patient's arm in front of the body with the arm laterally rotated so the medial aspect of the arm is visible.
2) Locate the medial epicondyle, then
3) Move distally just off the epicondyle to the joint space, staying posterior to the common flexor tendon.
4) The ligament is felt as a small band and can best be distinguished by moving back and forth across it.

● Ulnar Groove (Notch)

Skeletal and Anatomical Landmarks

Skeletal

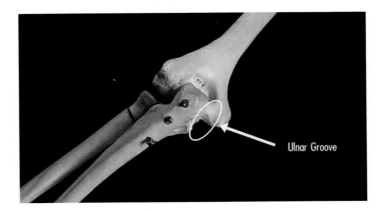

Anatomical

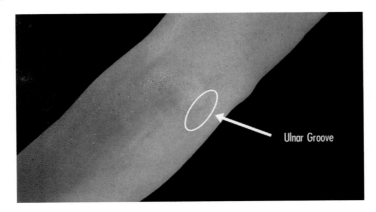

The ulnar groove is located on the medial, posterior aspect of the distal humerus. It houses the ulnar nerve as it passes the elbow.

Palpation Example

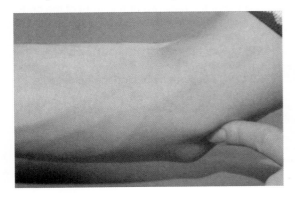

To palpate the ulnar groove,
1) Place the patient's arm in front of the body with the arm laterally rotated so the medial aspect of the arm is visible.
2) Locate the medial epicondyle of the humerus, then
3) Move posteriorly behind the epicondyle.
4) The ulnar groove is felt as a deep notch.

● Ulnar Nerve

Skeletal and Anatomical Landmarks

Skeletal

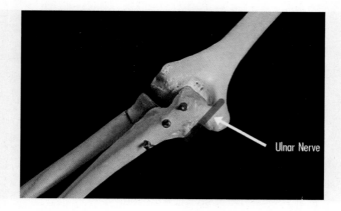

Anatomical

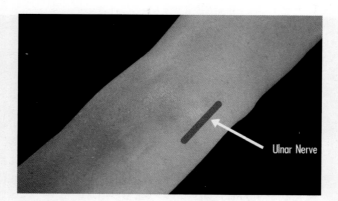

The ulnar nerve lies in the ulnar groove and runs through the medial forearm to the wrist.

Palpation Example

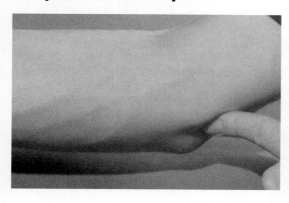

To palpate the ulnar nerve,
1) Place the patient's arm in front of the body with the arm laterally rotated so the medial aspect of the arm is visible.
2) Locate the medial epicondyle of the humerus, then
3) Move posteriorly behind the epicondyle into the ulnar groove.
4) Using the fingers, palpate along the ulnar groove.
5) The ulnar nerve lies deep in the groove.
6) Palpate gently because the nerve can be easily irritated.

● Triceps Tendon

Skeletal and Anatomical Landmarks

Skeletal

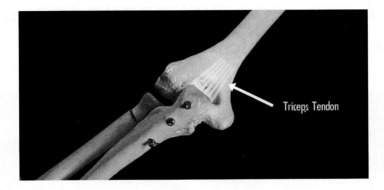

Anatomical

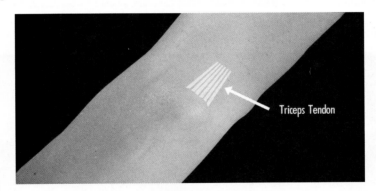

The triceps tendon is located on the posterior distal humerus and attaches to the olecranon process.

Palpation Example

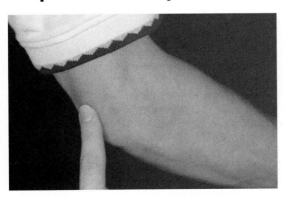

To palpate the triceps tendon,
1) Place the arm in front of the body with the elbow flexed and the arm internally rotated.
2) Ask the patient to try to extend the arm against slight resistance.
3) The triceps tendon becomes prominent and can be palpated as a thick band from the olecranon process about 3–4 inches up the posterior distal humerus.

⦿ Abductor Pollicis Longus Tendon

Skeletal and Anatomical Landmarks

Skeletal

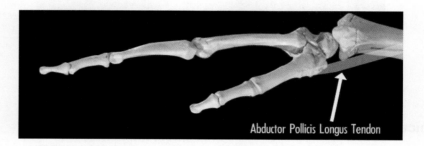

Abductor Pollicis Longus Tendon

Anatomical

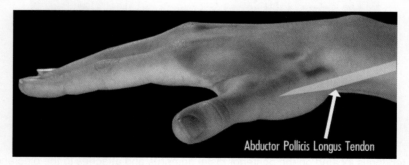

Abductor Pollicis Longus Tendon

The abductor pollicis longus tendon is the second tendon forming the ventral border of the anatomical snuffbox. It is slightly deeper and more anterior than the extensor pollicis brevis tendon.

Palpation Example

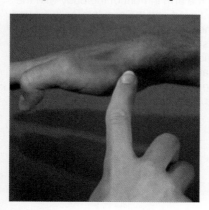

To palpate the abductor pollicis longus tendon,
1) Place the patient's hand in the neutral or slightly pronated position.
2) Ask the patient to extend and slightly abduct the thumb, exposing the anatomical snuffbox and its tendinous borders.
3) Locate the most prominent tendon of the ventral (palmar) border of the anatomical snuffbox (the extensor pollicis brevis tendon), then
4) Slide your finger toward the palm off the extensor pollicis brevis tendon. Another tendon should be felt immediately adjacent to the extensor pollicis brevis tendon and slightly deeper. That tendon is the abductor pollicis longus tendon.
5) The tendon can be palpated from the radial styloid to the 1st metacarpal.

● Anatomical Snuffbox

Skeletal and Anatomical Landmarks

Skeletal

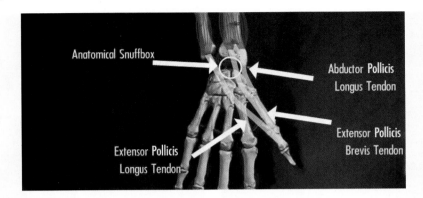

Anatomical

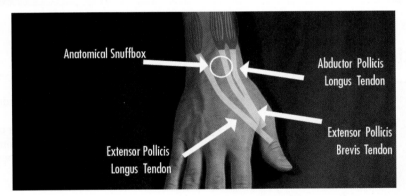

The anatomical snuffbox is the indentation formed when the thumb is extended. It is bordered by the extensor pollicis longus tendon on one side and the extensor pollicis brevis and abductor pollicis longus tendons on the other.

Palpation Example

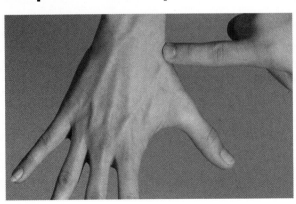

To palpate the anatomical snuffbox,
1) Place the patient's hand in the neutral or pronated position.
2) Ask the patient to extend the thumb. A large divot becomes visible on the lateral wrist just distal to the radial styloid.
3) The divot, called the anatomical snuffbox, is created by the tendons that extend and/or abduct the thumb.
4) Palpate deep in the indentation between the tendons.

◉ Capitate

Skeletal and Anatomical Landmarks

Skeletal   **Anatomical**

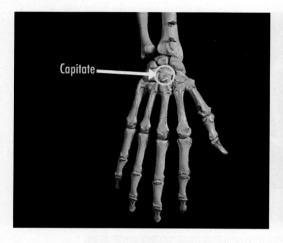   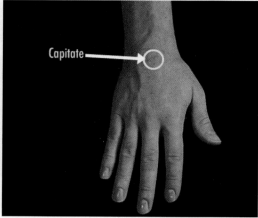

The capitate is located in the distal row of carpals, just proximal to the 3rd metacarpal.

Palpation Example

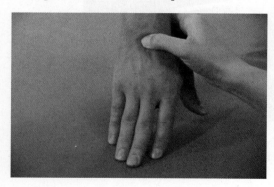

To palpate the capitate,
1) Place the patient's wrist in the pronated position.
2) Locate the 3rd metacarpal and move proximally until you feel the divot proximal to the metacarpal and distal to the radius.
3) Press into the divot.
4) The capitate forms the floor of this depression.

TIP

Flexing the Wrist

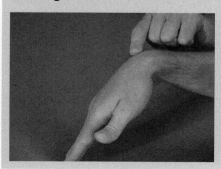

The capitate will protrude slightly when the wrist is flexed and recess, creating a divot, when the wrist is extended.

◉ Distal Interphalangeal Joints (Hand)

Skeletal and Anatomical Landmarks

Skeletal

Anatomical

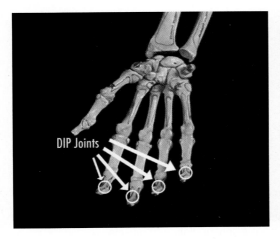

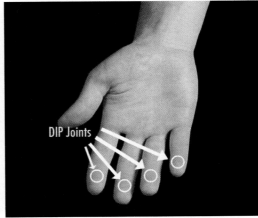

The distal interphalangeal (DIP) joints are the distal-most joints of fingers 2–5.

Palpation Example

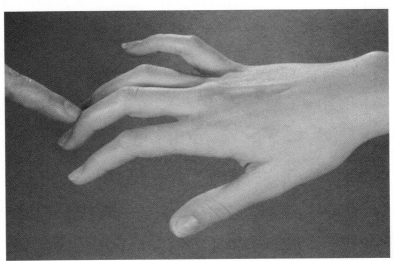

To palpate the DIP joints of the fingers,
1) Place the hand in an open position with the fingers extended.
2) Locate the most distal joint on fingers 2–5.
3) The joints can be palpated with a single digit or by pinching the joint gently between the finger and thumb.
4) The joints should be palpated on all sides.

◉ Extensor Carpi Radialis Muscle

Skeletal and Anatomical Landmarks

Skeletal

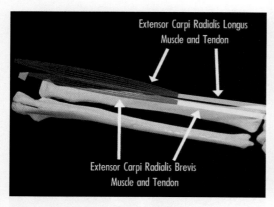

Anatomical

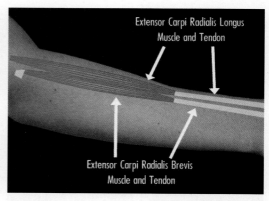

The extensor carpi radialis longus and brevis muscles are located on the proximal posterior forearm, medial to the brachioradialis and lateral to the extensor digitorum muscle.

Palpation Example

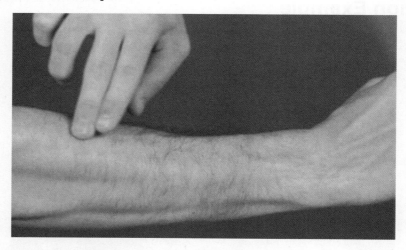

To palpate the extensor carpi radialis longus and brevis muscles,
1) Place the patient's arm in the neutral or pronated position.
2) Locate the brachioradialis muscle then move medially on the posterior forearm just off the brachioradialis muscle to the next palpable muscle belly.
3) That muscle group should be the extensor carpi radialis longus and brevis muscle bellies.
4) To verify that you are on the correct muscles, ask the patient to extend the wrist against slight resistance.
5) The muscle bellies should become more prominent under your fingers.
6) If you are too far medially, you will be on the extensor digitorum muscle, which can be verified by having the patient extend the fingers against resistance and feeling for the muscle to become more prominent.

⦿ Extensor Carpi Radialis Tendon

Skeletal and Anatomical Landmarks

Skeletal

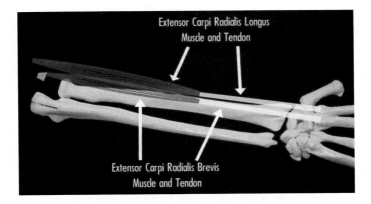

Anatomical

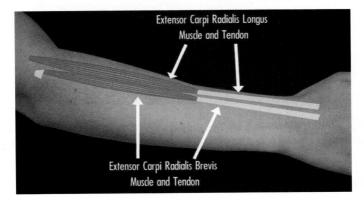

The extensor carpi radialis longus and brevis tendons are located between the extensor indices tendon and the extensor pollicis longus tendon. They insert on the bases of the 2nd and 3rd metacarpals.

Palpation Example

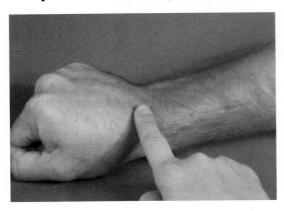

To palpate the extensor carpi radialis longus and brevis tendons,

1) Place the patient's forearm in the neutral or pronated position.
2) Ask the patient to squeeze the hand to a fist and slightly extend the wrist.
3) A larger tendon bundle (the extensor carpi radialis longus and brevis tendons) will become prominent medial to the extensor pollicis longus tendon of the anatomical snuffbox and lateral to the extensor indices tendon where it crosses the wrist.
4) The tendon can be palpated a couple of inches in length.

● Extensor Carpi Ulnaris Muscle

Skeletal and Anatomical Landmarks

Skeletal

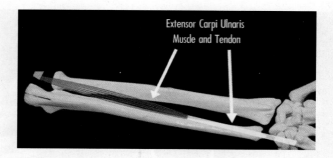

Anatomical

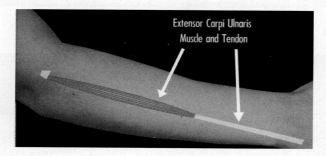

The extensor carpi ulnaris muscle lies on the medial side of the posterior forearm. It originates on the lateral epicondyle via the common extensor tendon and inserts on the base of the 5th metacarpal.

Palpation Example

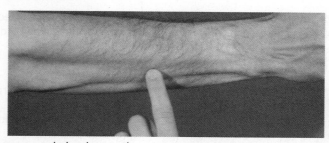

To palpate the extensor carpi ulnaris muscle,
1) Place the patient's forearm in the pronated position.
2) While palpating the posterior proximal forearm just lateral to the bony ridge of the ulna, ask the patient to extend and ulnarly deviate the wrist against slight resistance.
3) The extensor carpi ulnaris muscle will be felt contracting under your fingers.
4) The muscle lies medial to the extensor digitorum muscle, so you can verify your placement by moving laterally to the next muscle belly and confirming that muscle's identity by asking the patient to extend the fingers against resistance.
5) The extensor carpi ulnaris muscle can be palpated for several inches from the mid forearm to its proximal attachment on the lateral epicondyle.

⦿ Extensor Carpi Ulnaris Tendon

Skeletal and Anatomical Landmarks

Skeletal

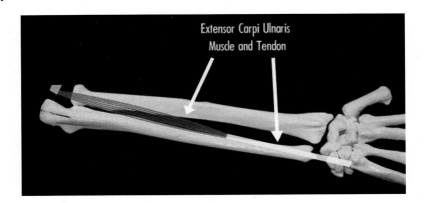

Anatomical

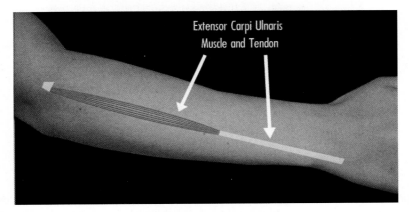

The extensor carpi ulnaris tendon is located on the posterior medial aspect of the forearm. It runs medial to the ulnar styloid and inserts on the base of the 5th metacarpal.

Palpation Example

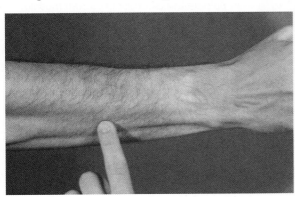

To palpate the extensor carpi ulnaris tendon,
1) Place the patient's forearm in the pronated position.
2) Ask the patient to slightly extend and ulnarly deviate the wrist.
3) Locate the tendon that becomes visible and palpable along the medial posterior forearm, medial to the ulnar styloid and lateral to the bony ridge of the ulna.
4) The tendon can be palpated for a few inches along the forearm.

◉ Extensor Digitorum Muscle

Skeletal and Anatomical Landmarks

Skeletal

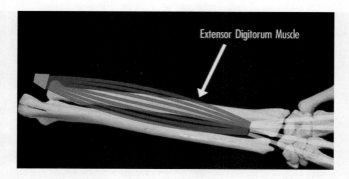

Anatomical

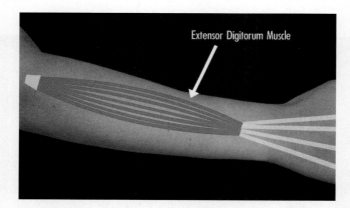

The extensor digitorum muscle lies on the middle of the posterior forearm. It originates on the lateral epicondyle via the common extensor tendon and splits into four tendons on the distal end to insert on the distal phalanges of digits 2–5.

Palpation Example

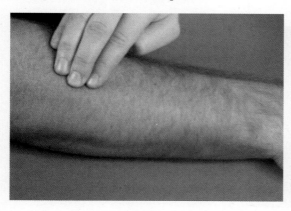

To palpate the extensor digitorum muscle,
1) Place the patient's forearm in the neutral or pronated position.
2) Locate the broader muscle near the midline of the posterior proximal forearm, medial to the extensor carpi radialis longus and brevis muscles and lateral to the extensor carpi ulnaris muscle.
3) To verify that you are on the correct muscle, ask the patient to extend the fingers against slight resistance.
4) The muscle will be felt contracting under your fingers if you are on the correct structure.

◉ Extensor Digitorum Tendons

Skeletal and Anatomical Landmarks

Skeletal

Anatomical

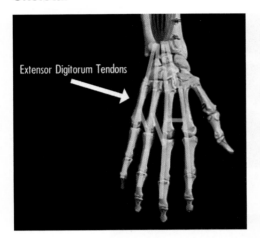

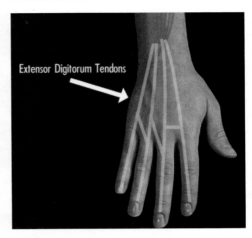

The extensor digitorum tendons are located on the posterior aspect of the hand. They are easily visible and palpable.

Palpation Example

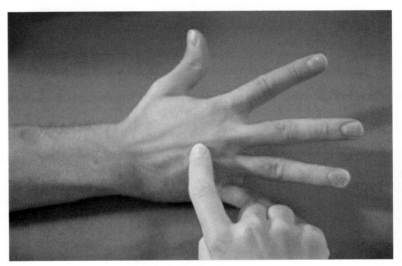

To palpate the extensor digitorum tendons,
1) Place the patient's hand in the pronated position.
2) Ask the patient to extend the fingers against slight resistance.
3) Locate the tendons that become visible and palpable on the dorsal aspect of the hand.
4) The tendons can be traced along the dorsum of the hand from the phalanges of fingers 2–5 to the wrist.

◉ Extensor Pollicis Brevis Tendon

Skeletal and Anatomical Landmarks

Skeletal

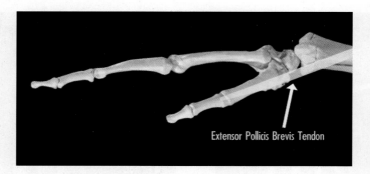

Extensor Pollicis Brevis Tendon

Anatomical

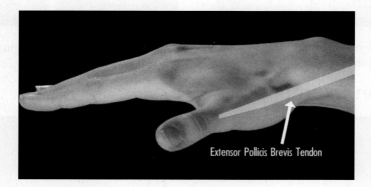

Extensor Pollicis Brevis Tendon

The extensor pollicis brevis tendon forms the ventral border of the anatomical snuffbox.

Palpation Example

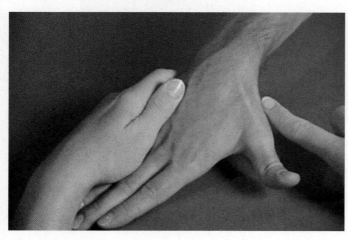

To palpate the extensor pollicis brevis tendon,

1) Place the patient's hand in the neutral or pronated position.
2) Ask the patient to extend the thumb, exposing the anatomical snuffbox.
3) The tendon that forms the ventral border of the anatomical snuffbox is the extensor pollicis brevis tendon.
4) The tendon can be palpated from the radial styloid to the proximal phalanx of the thumb.

● Extensor Pollicis Longus Tendon

Skeletal and Anatomical Landmarks

Skeletal

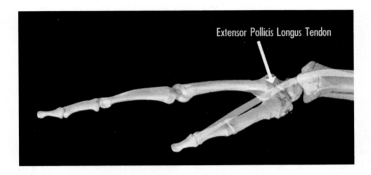

Extensor Pollicis Longus Tendon

Anatomical

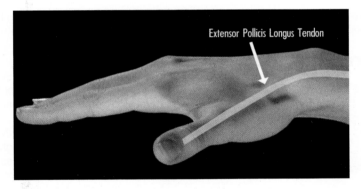

Extensor Pollicis Longus Tendon

The extensor pollicis longus tendon is the most dorsal tendon of the anatomical snuffbox. It extends from the wrist to the distal phalanx of the thumb.

Palpation Example

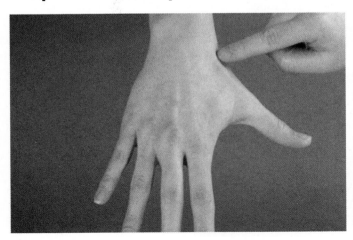

To palpate the extensor pollicis longus tendon,

1) Place the patient's hand in the neutral or pronated position.
2) Ask the patient to extend the thumb, exposing the anatomical snuffbox.
3) The tendon that forms the dorsal border of the anatomical snuffbox is the extensor pollicis longus tendon.
4) The tendon can be palpated from the radial styloid to the distal phalanx of the thumb.

◉ Flexor Carpi Radialis Tendon

Skeletal and Anatomical Landmarks

Skeletal   **Anatomical**

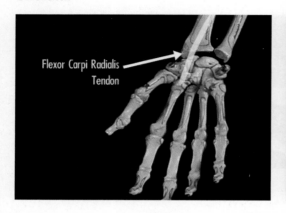

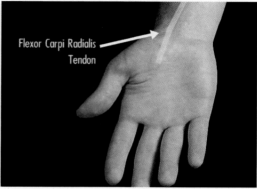

The flexor carpi radialis tendon runs along the anterior aspect of the wrist lateral to the palmaris longus. It attaches to the bases of the 2nd and 3rd metacarpals.

Palpation Example

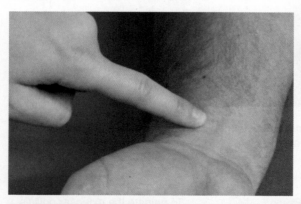

To palpate the flexor carpi radialis tendon,
1) Place the patient's wrist in the neutral or supinated position.
2) Ask the patient to gently flex the wrist against resistance. Slight radial deviation may also be necessary to make the tendon more prominent.
3) Locate the tendon that is proximal to the thenar eminence and lateral to the palmaris longus tendon.
4) This tendon is the flexor carpi radialis tendon. It can be palpated 3–4 inches up the forearm.

TIP

Clench Fist or Flex Wrist

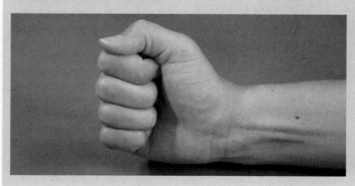

The flexor carpi radialis tendon can be palpated by asking the patient to clench the fist and/or flex the wrist.

● Flexor Carpi Ulnaris Tendon

Skeletal and Anatomical Landmarks

Skeletal   **Anatomical**

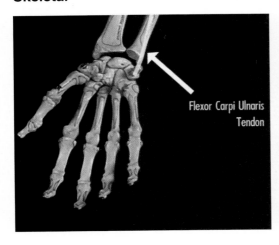

Flexor Carpi Ulnaris
Tendon

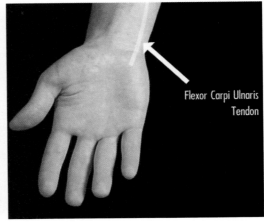

Flexor Carpi Ulnaris
Tendon

The flexor carpi ulnaris tendon runs along the anterior medial aspect of the wrist and attaches to the pisiform.

Palpation Example

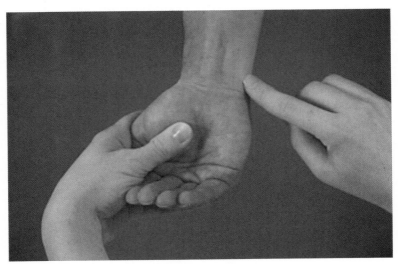

To palpate the flexor carpi ulnaris tendon,
1) Place the patient's wrist in the supinated position.
2) Ask the patient to gently flex the wrist against resistance. Slight ulnar deviation may also be necessary to make the tendon more prominent.
3) Locate the tendon that is proximal to the pisiform.
4) This tendon is the flexor carpi ulnaris tendon. It can be palpated 2–3 inches up the forearm.

Flexor Digitorum Profundus Tendons

Skeletal and Anatomical Landmarks

Skeletal

Anatomical

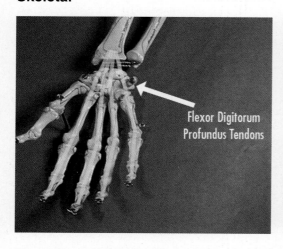

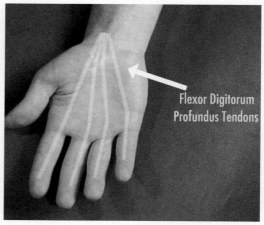

The tendons of flexor digitorum profundus cross the anterior aspect of the proximal and distal interphalangeal joints (PIP and DIP joints) and insert on the distal phalanx.

Palpation Example

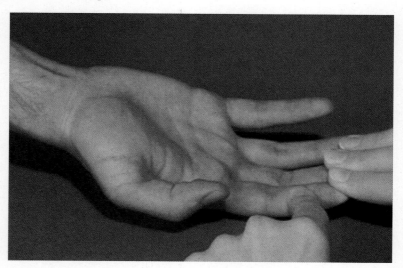

To palpate the flexor digitorum profundus tendons,
1) Place the patient's hand in the supinated position.
2) While holding the distal phalanx with one hand, ask the patient to flex the fingers against slight resistance.
3) Use the index finger or thumb of your other hand to locate the tendons that become prominent on the palmar surface just proximal to the crease of the DIP joints of fingers 2–5.

Flexor Digitorum Superficialis Tendons

Skeletal and Anatomical Landmarks

Skeletal

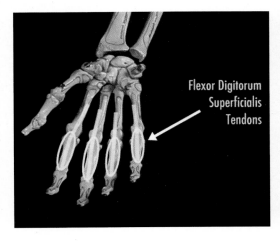

Flexor Digitorum
Superficialis
Tendons

Anatomical

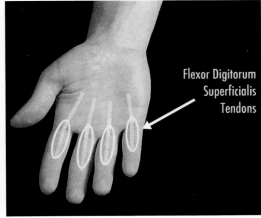

Flexor Digitorum
Superficialis
Tendons

The tendons of flexor digitorum superficialis cross the anterior aspect of the PIP joints and insert on the middle phalanx.

Palpation Example

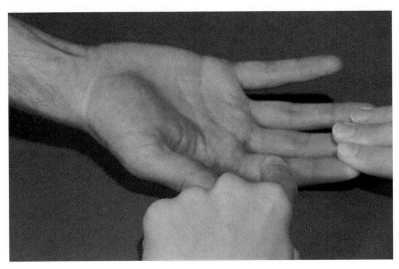

To palpate the flexor digitorum superficialis tendons,
1) Place the patient's hand in the supinated position.
2) While holding the middle phalanx with one hand, ask the patient to flex the fingers against slight resistance.
3) Use the index finger or thumb of your other hand to locate the tendons that become prominent on the palmar surface at the crease of the PIP joints of fingers 2 to 5.

◉ Heads of the Metacarpals

Skeletal and Anatomical Landmarks

Skeletal   **Anatomical**

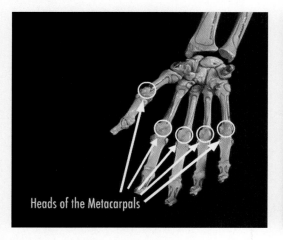

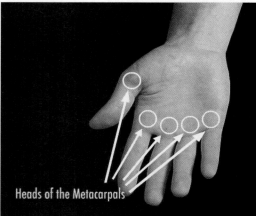

The head of the metacarpal is the distal end of the metacarpal.

Palpation Example

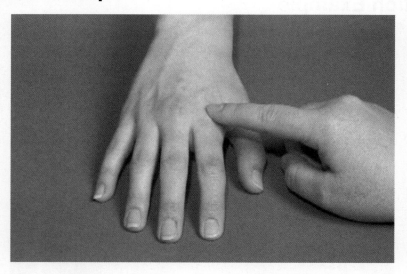

To palpate the head of each metacarpal,

1) Place the patient's hand in either the supinated or pronated position, depending on the location of the intended palpation.
2) Locate what is commonly referred to as the ball of the hand or the first knuckle.
3) The head of the metacarpal is the proximal portion of that area.
4) Using your thumb, one finger, or by holding the metacarpal head between your thumb and index finger, palpate the full circumference of the bone.

◉ Hook of the Hamate

Skeletal and Anatomical Landmarks

Skeletal

Anatomical

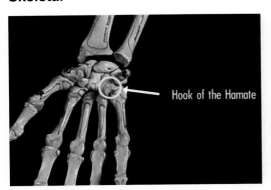

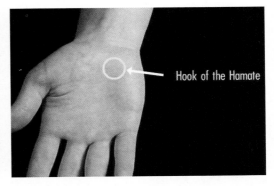

The hook of the hamate is located beneath the center of the proximal half of the hypothenar eminence. The hook of the hamate forms the lateral border of the Tunnel of Guyon.

Palpation Example

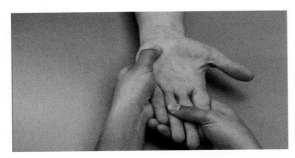

To palpate the hook of the hamate,
1) Place the patient's hand in supinated position.
2) Locate the pisiform, then
3) Move approximately one to one and a half inches toward the base of the index finger.
4) The hook of the hamate is felt as a small "ball" in the center of the proximal aspect of the hypothenar eminence.
5) Pressure in this area may cause the patient to withdraw.

Alternate View

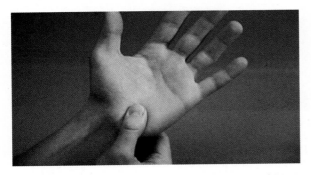

To palpate the hook of the hamate using an alternate method,
1) Locate the pisiform, then
2) Place the interphalangeal joint of your thumb on the pisiform.
3) Point your thumb toward the base of the index finger and rest the tip of your thumb on the patient's palm.
4) The hook of the hamate lies just below the distal aspect of your thumb and can be felt as a small ball.

TIP

Patient Pulls Back
The region over the hook of the hamate may be tender. Pressure in this area may cause the patient to withdraw.

⦿ Hypothenar Eminence

Skeletal and Anatomical Landmarks

Skeletal

Anatomical

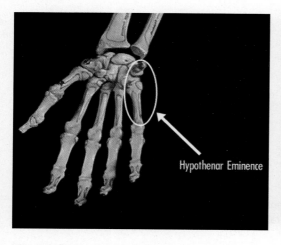

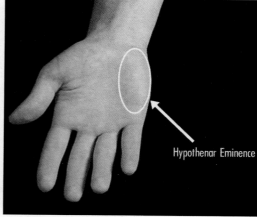

The hypothenar eminence is the group of muscles creating the padlike appearance on the medial (pinky) side of the palm.

Palpation Example

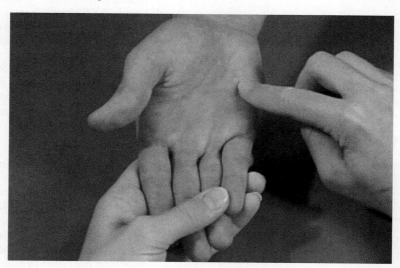

To palpate the hypothenar eminence,
1) Place the patient's hand in the supinated position.
2) Locate the padlike structure on the medial aspect of the palm, over the 5th metacarpal region.
3) This muscle bundle is the hypothenar eminence.

Lister's Tubercle

Skeletal and Anatomical Landmarks

Skeletal   **Anatomical**

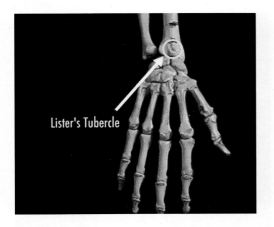

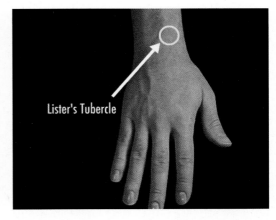

Lister's tubercle is a small bony prominence that lies on the dorsum of the radius approximately ⅓ of the way between the radial and ulnar styloids. Lister's tubercle lies proximal to the lunate and directly in line with the 3rd metacarpal, the capitate, and the lunate.

Palpation Example

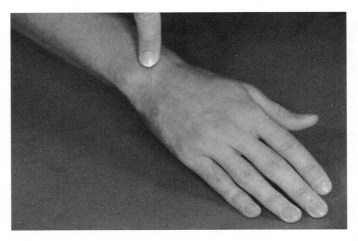

To palpate Lister's tubercle,
1) Place the patient's hand in the pronated position.
2) Locate the divot of the capitate, then
3) Move proximally past the lunate and onto the radius.
4) Lister's tubercle will be felt as a smaller, pointed bone on the distal radius between the radial and ulnar styloid processes.

Alternate Method:
To palpate Lister's tubercle,
1) Start from the radial styloid.
2) Move approximately ⅓ of the way across the dorsum of the wrist toward the ulnar styloid.
3) Lister's tubercle will be felt as a smaller, pointed bone.

◉ Lunate

Skeletal and Anatomical Landmarks

Skeletal   **Anatomical**

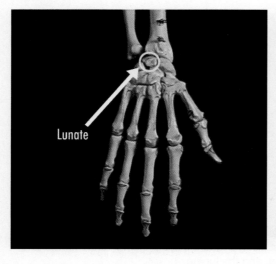

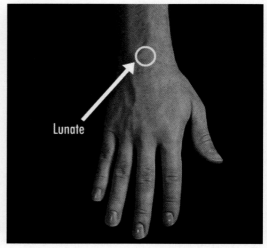

The lunate is the carpal bone that lies proximal to the capitate.

Palpation Example

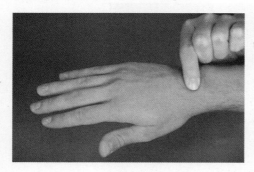

To palpate the lunate,
1) Place the patient's hand in the pronated position.
2) Locate the 3rd metacarpal, then
3) Move proximally into the divot that contains the capitate.
4) From this depression, move proximally onto a small ridge of bone that acts as the proximal border to the capitate depression.
5) The lunate becomes more prominent when the wrist is flexed.

TIP

Flex Wrist

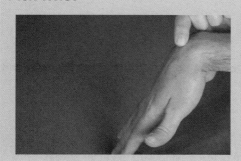

The lunate becomes more prominent when the wrist is flexed.

● Metacarpal-Phalangeal Joints

Skeletal and Anatomical Landmarks

Skeletal

Anatomical

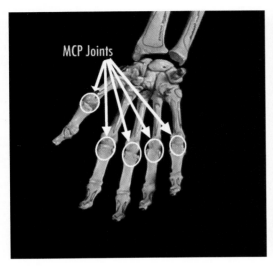 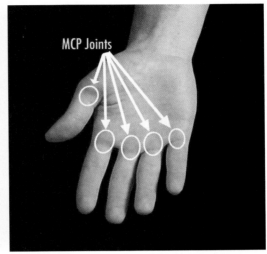

The metacarpal-phalangeal joints (MCP joints) are the joints between the palm of the hand and the fingers or thumb.

Palpation Example

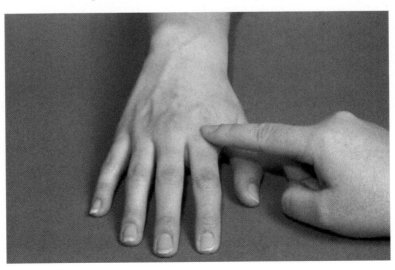

To palpate the MCP joints,
1) Place the patient's hand in either the pronated or supinated position, depending on the location of the pain or injury.
2) Locate what is commonly referred to as the balls of the hand or the first knuckles where the fingers and thumb meet the hand.
3) The MCP joints lie at the center of those areas.

⦿ Metacarpals

Skeletal and Anatomical Landmarks

Skeletal   **Anatomical**

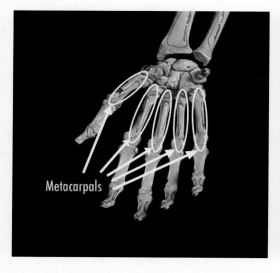   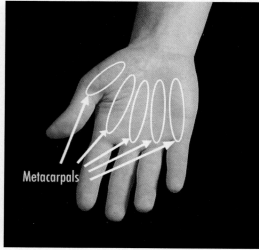

The metacarpals are the long bones in the palm of the hand proximal to the fingers and thumb.

Palpation Example

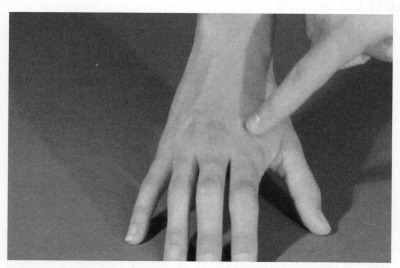

To palpate the metacarpals,
1) Place the patient's hand in the pronated position.
2) Locate the long bones on the dorsum of the palm.
3) They are directly proximal to each finger and thumb and extend approximately ⅔ of the way to the wrist.

◉ Palmaris Longus Tendon

Skeletal and Anatomical Landmarks

Skeletal	Anatomical

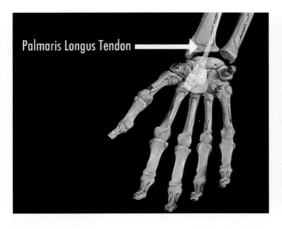

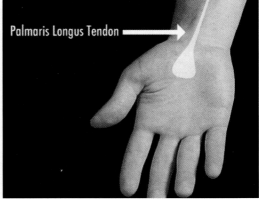

The palmaris longus tendon lies medial to the flexor carpi radialis tendon and attaches to the palmar aponeurosis.

Palpation Example

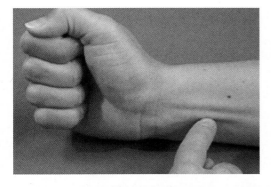

To palpate the palmaris longus tendon,
1) Place the patient's hand in the supinated position.
2) Ask the patient to touch the thumb and fingers together then slightly flex the wrist.
3) Sometimes, the tendon will also become prominent by asking the patient to simply clench the fist.
4) Locate the broader palmaris longus tendon as it lies along the midline of the anterior aspect of the wrist, remembering that some patients may not have this tendon.

TIP

Touching Thumb and Fingers

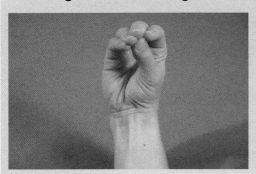

The palmaris longus tendon is best palpated by asking the patient to touch the thumb and fingers together then flex the wrist.

◉ Phalanges (Hand)

Skeletal and Anatomical Landmarks

Skeletal   **Anatomical**

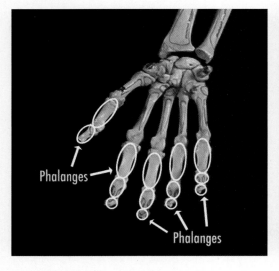   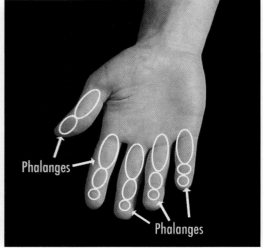

The phalanges of the hand are the bones of the fingers.

Palpation Example

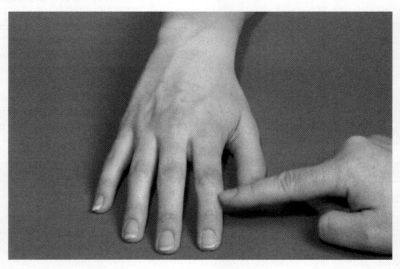

To palpate the phalanges of the hand,

1) Place the patient's hand in the pronated or supinated position, depending on the location of the injury.
2) Locate each segment of the fingers, remembering there are only two phalanges in the thumb and three in each of the other fingers.
3) The phalanges can be palpated with a single finger or by gently pinching the bones between your thumb and fingers.

◉ Pisiform

Skeletal and Anatomical Landmarks

Skeletal   **Anatomical**

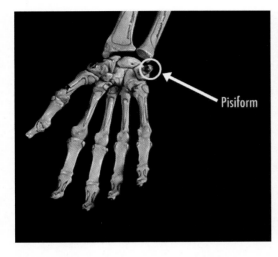

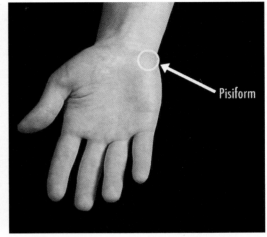

The pisiform is located on the palmar aspect of the wrist. It is the medial-most bone in the proximal row of carpals.

Palpation Example

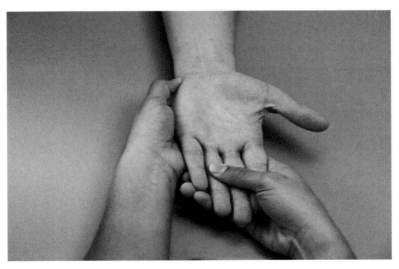

To palpate the pisiform,
1) Place the patient's hand in the supinated position.
2) Locate the small, ball-like bone located at the proximal, medial corner of the hand where the hypothenar eminence and the crease of the wrist meet.

◉ Proximal Interphalangeal Joints (Hand)

Skeletal and Anatomical Landmarks

Skeletal   **Anatomical**

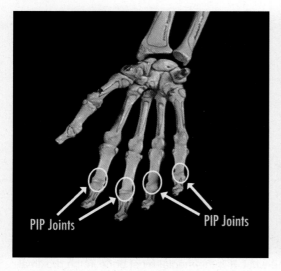 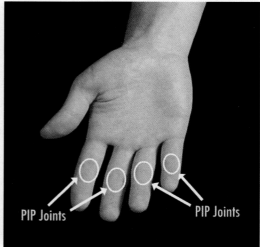

The PIP joint is the most proximal joint of the two joints in fingers 2–5.

Palpation Example

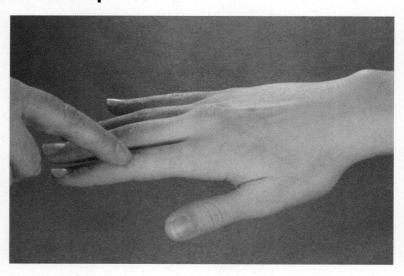

To palpate the PIP joints of the hand,
1) Place the patient's hand in the pronated or supinated position, depending on the location of the injury.
2) Locate the most proximal joint of the two interphalangeal joints of fingers 2–5.
3) The joints can be palpated with a single finger or by gently pinching the joints between your thumb and fingers.

⦿ Radial Pulse

Skeletal and Anatomical Landmarks

Skeletal   **Anatomical**

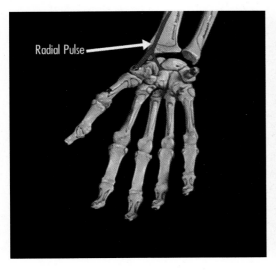   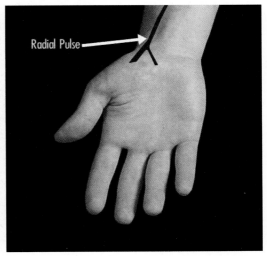

The radial pulse is located on the lateral aspect of the anterior wrist.

Palpation Example

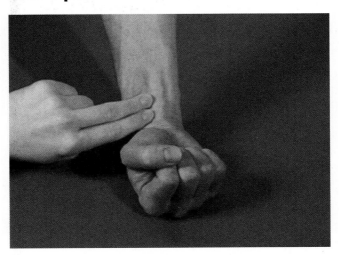

To palpate the radial pulse,
1) Place the patient in a seated position at the end of the treatment table with the hand supinated, exposing the anterior aspect of the wrist.
2) Place your index and middle fingers on the wrist one or two finger widths proximal to the thenar eminence and just lateral to the flexor carpi radialis tendon.
3) Gentle pressure will enable easier palpation of the pulse.

◉ Radial Styloid

Skeletal and Anatomical Landmarks

Skeletal

Anatomical

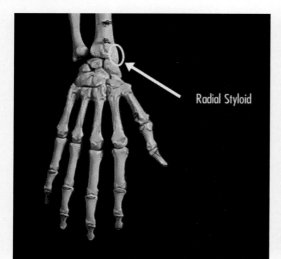

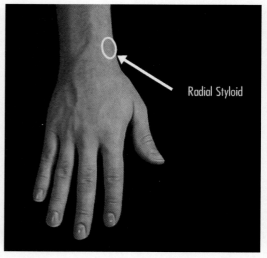

The radial styloid is located on the distal radius, proximal to the scaphoid.

Palpation Example

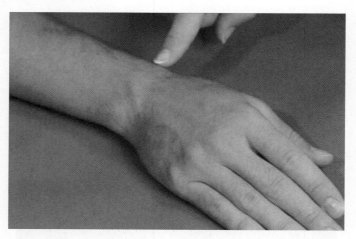

To palpate the radial styloid,
1) Place the patient's hand in the pronated or neutral position. The patient may be seated at the end of the treatment table or standing.
2) Locate the anatomical snuffbox, then
3) Move proximally one or two finger widths to the large bony prominence on the lateral distal radius.
4) This bony prominence is the radial styloid.
5) The extensor pollicis brevis tendon is also in direct line with the radial styloid and can be used as a reference point to locate the bone.

● Scaphoid

Skeletal and Anatomical Landmarks

Skeletal

Anatomical

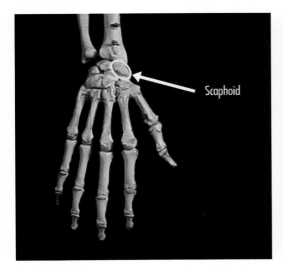

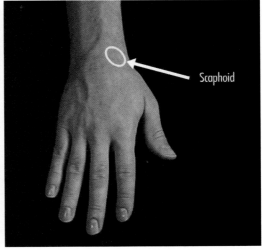

The scaphoid lies distal to the radius and is the lateral-most carpal bone in the proximal row of carpals. It makes up the floor of the anatomical snuffbox.

Palpation Example

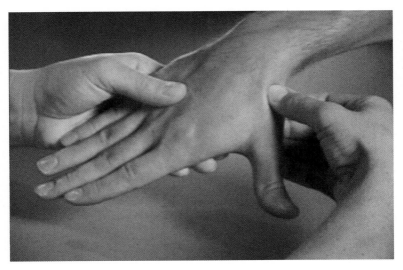

To palpate the scaphoid,
1) Place the patient's hand in the pronated or neutral position in front of the body.
2) Ask the patient to extend the thumb, exposing the anatomical snuffbox.
3) Because the scaphoid makes up the floor of the anatomical snuffbox, press straight into the snuffbox toward its floor.
4) The scaphoid becomes more prominent when the wrist is ulnarly deviated.

◉ Thenar Eminence

Skeletal and Anatomical Landmarks

Skeletal   **Anatomical**

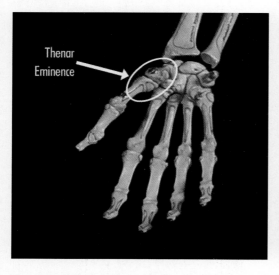 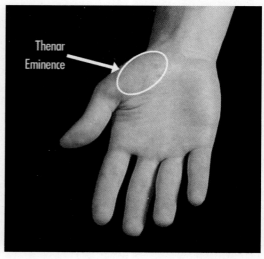

The thenar eminence is the group of muscles creating the padlike appearance on the lateral side of the palm, proximal to the thumb.

Palpation Example

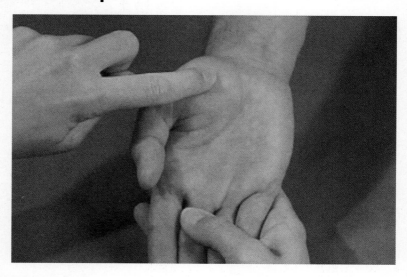

To palpate the thenar eminence,
1) Place the patient's hand in the supinated position.
2) Locate the padlike structure on the lateral aspect of the palm, over the 1st metacarpal region.
3) Palpate the full width and length of the thenar eminence.

Trapezium

Skeletal and Anatomical Landmarks

Skeletal

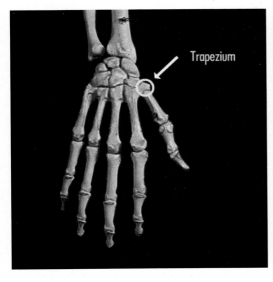

Anatomical

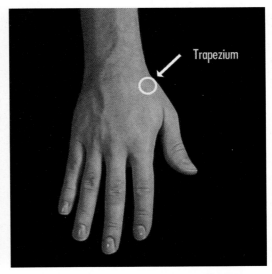

The trapezium is the lateral-most bone in the distal row of carpals. It lies distal to the scaphoid and proximal to the 1st metacarpal.

Palpation Example

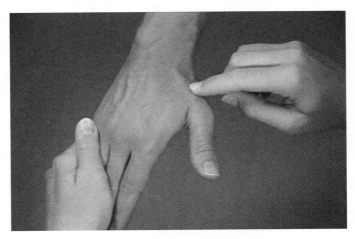

To palpate the trapezium,
1) Place the patient's hand in the pronated position.
2) Locate the anatomical snuffbox and place your finger in the snuffbox.
3) From there, move just distal to the snuffbox onto the next bone (the trapezium), which forms the distal wall of the snuffbox.
4) Flexing and extending the thumb may help to locate the bone as the evaluator feels for joint motion between the bones.

◉ Trapezoid

Skeletal and Anatomical Landmarks

Skeletal   **Anatomical**

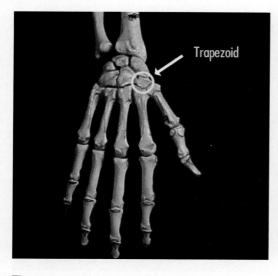

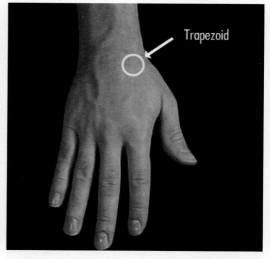

The trapezoid is the small carpal bone that lies proximal to the 2nd metacarpal and medial to the trapezium.

Palpation Example

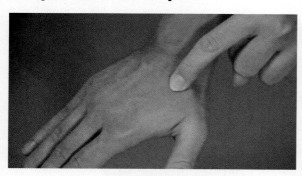

To palpate the trapezoid,
1) Place the patient's hand in the pronated position.
2) Locate the 2nd metacarpal, then
3) Move proximally into the divot located proximal to the metacarpal.
4) The trapezoid lies in this divot.

Alternate Method

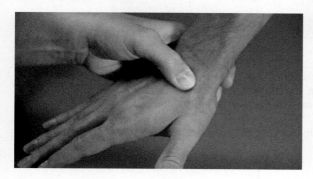

Alternate Method:
1) You can also locate the trapezoid by locating the anatomical snuffbox, then
2) Jump over the extensor pollicis longus tendon to a small divot that is in line with the 2nd metacarpal.
3) The trapezoid lies in this divot.

Triquetrum

Skeletal and Anatomical Landmarks

Skeletal

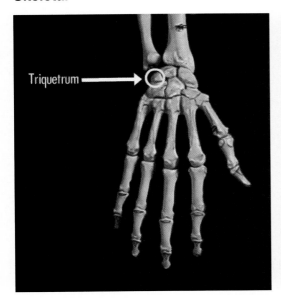

Anatomical

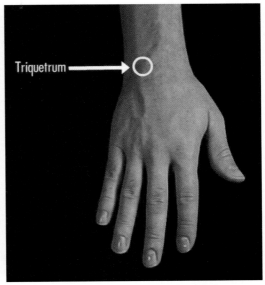

The triquetrum is located on the medial aspect of the wrist in the proximal row of carpals. It lies posterior to the pisiform.

Palpation Example

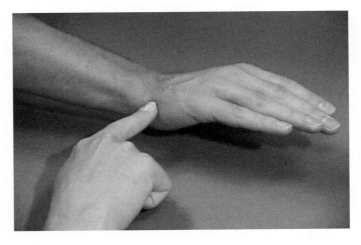

To palpate the triquetrum,
1) Place the patient's hand in the pronated position.
2) Place one finger on the medial aspect of the wrist (pinky side) at the crease between the hand and the forearm, medial to the pisiform and distal to the ulnar styloid.
3) The triquetrum is located in this crease and can be felt protruding and retracting as the wrist is radially and ulnarly deviated.

⦿ Ulnar Pulse

Skeletal and Anatomical Landmarks

Skeletal

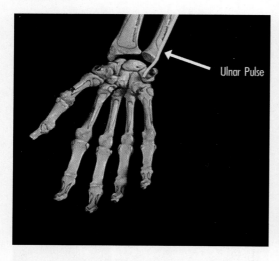

Anatomical

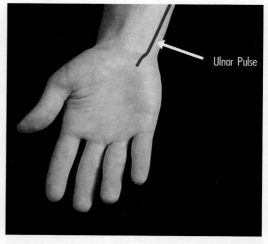

The ulnar artery extends down the anterior medial forearm and is palpable lateral to the flexor carpi ulnaris tendon at the wrist.

Palpation Example

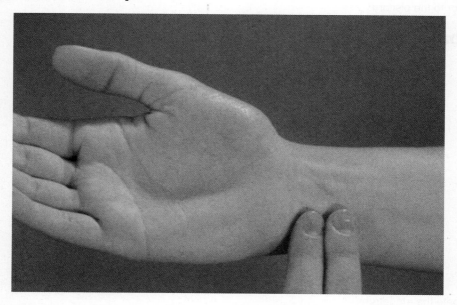

To palpate the ulnar pulse,
1) Place the patient's hand in the supinated position.
2) Place your index and middle fingers lateral to the flexor carpi ulnaris tendon just proximal to the crease of the wrist.
3) Gentle pressure will enable easier palpation of the pulse.

◉ Ulnar Styloid

Skeletal and Anatomical Landmarks

Skeletal

Anatomical

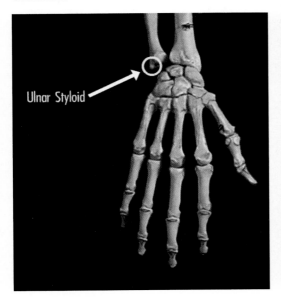
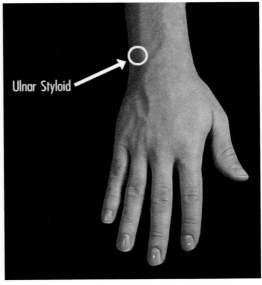

The ulnar styloid is the large bony protrusion on the medial dorsum of the wrist.

Palpation Example

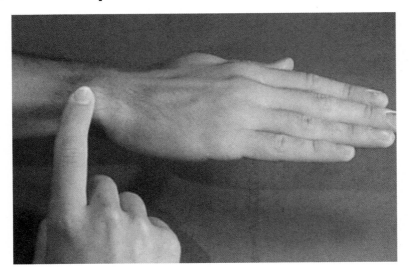

To palpate the ulnar styloid,
1) Place the patient's hand in the pronated position.
2) Locate the large bony protrusion on the medial (pinky side) dorsum of the wrist.
3) Move distally just off that protrusion.
4) The ulnar styloid lies deep to your finger at the edge of the larger protrusion.

SECTION II

Lower Body Palpations

● Adductor Longus Muscle

Skeletal and Anatomical Landmarks

Skeletal

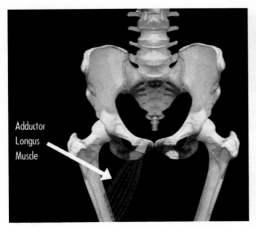

Anatomical

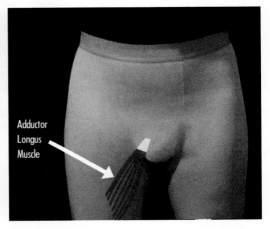

The adductor longus muscle originates on the pubic tubercle. It is the anterior/lateral of the two prominent tendons originating from the pubic tubercles.

Palpation Example

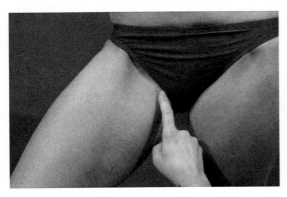

To palpate the adductor longus tendon,
1) Place the patient in the supine position. Stand to the side of the patient.
2) Ask the patient to slightly flex and externally rotate the hip.
3) Two large tendons will become prominent on the superior thigh just distal to the pubic tubercle. The adductor longus tendon is the more anterior and lateral of the two tendons.
4) The tendon can be palpated from the pubic tubercle distally for 3–4 inches.
5) If the tendon is difficult to distinguish, ask the patient to rotate the thigh medially and laterally while flexed. The tendon should become very prominent as the thigh moves.

⬤ Anterior Superior Iliac Spine

Skeletal and Anatomical Landmarks

Skeletal

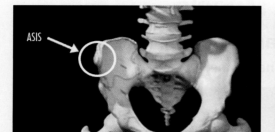

Anatomical

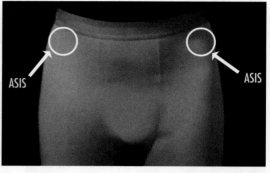

The ASIS (anterior superior iliac spine) is the anterior-most aspect of the iliac bone. It is the most prominent bone on the anterior, superior, lateral aspect of the pelvis.

Palpation Example

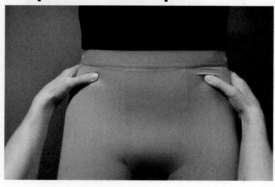

To palpate the ASIS,
1) Place the patient either standing or lying in a supine position.
2) To palpate the ASIS of a patient who is standing, place your hands on the sides of the patient's waist on the iliac crests (bony ridges), then
3) Rest your thumbs down on the front of the body, inferior to the iliac crests.
4) The ASIS are the most bony prominences on the front of the pelvis just inferior to the waistline. They can be specifically located by moving the thumbs in a circular motion.

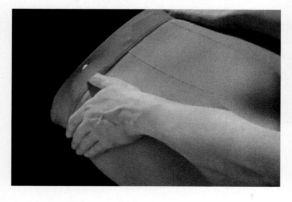

Locating the ASIS on patients with larger body masses and/or less prominent bones can be difficult. To palpate the ASIS of a patient who is in the supine position,
1) Place the palm of your hand on the anterior lateral pelvic region of the patient just below the waistband. (You may have to press down or move your hand back and forth slightly).
2) The ASIS should be felt as the most prominent bony protrusion under the palm.
3) You can then slide your hand off the landmark and palpate the ASIS with your thumb or fingers.

◉ Coccyx

Skeletal and Anatomical Landmarks

Skeletal

Anatomical

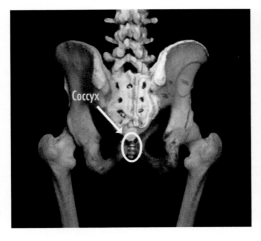

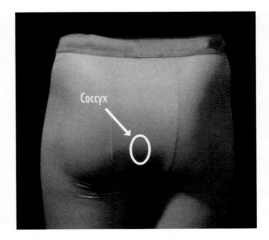

The coccyx, often referred to as the tailbone, lies just distal to the sacrum.

Palpation Example

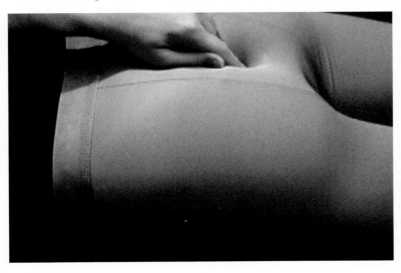

To palpate the coccyx,
1) Place the patient in the prone position on the treatment table.
2) Locate the sacrum, then move distally along the sacrum until a bony drop-off is felt.
3) The coccyx is located about one finger width distal to the drop-off (at the upper edge of the gluteal crease).
4) Use caution when palpating the coccyx because excess pressure can cause injury.

● Gluteus Maximus Muscle

Skeletal and Anatomical Landmarks

Skeletal   **Anatomical**

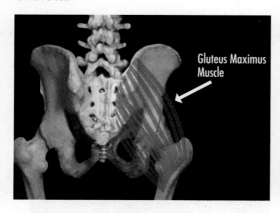 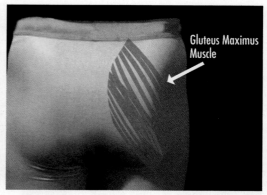

The gluteus maximus is the large muscle of the buttocks. It arises from the posterior upper ilium and sacrum and inserts on the IT band and lateral ridge of the linea aspera (gluteal tuberosity) of the femur.

Palpation Example

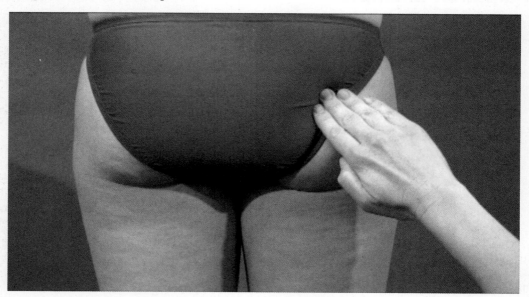

To palpate the gluteus maximus muscle,
1) Place the patient in prone position on the treatment table or in a standing position.
2) Locate the large muscle mass of the buttock.
3) Palpate the muscle in a diagonal direction from the posterior iliac crest and sacrum to the upper femur.

● Gluteus Medius Muscle

Skeletal and Anatomical Landmarks

Skeletal   **Anatomical**

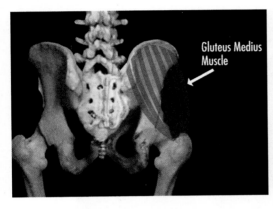

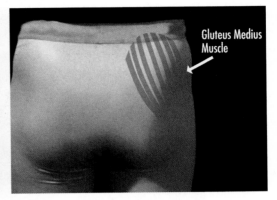

The gluteus medius muscle lies partially under the gluteus maximus. It arises from the outer, upper surface of the iliac crest and inserts on the lateral surface of the greater trochanter.

Palpation Example

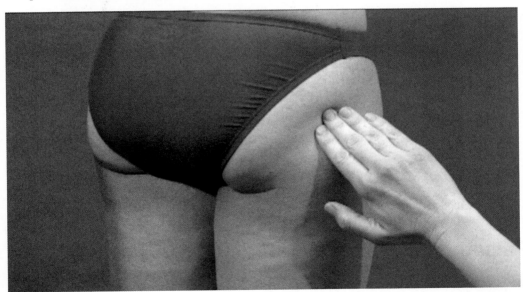

To palpate the gluteus medius muscle,
1) Place the patient in a prone or standing position.
2) Locate the region inferior to the iliac crest, anterior to the gluteus maximus muscle and posterior to the tensor facia lata muscle. The gluteus medius muscle lies in this area.
3) The muscle will become more palpable if the patient can abduct the leg against slight resistance.

◉ Gracilis Tendon/Muscle

Skeletal and Anatomical Landmarks

Skeletal

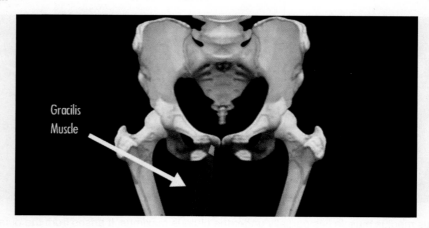

Gracilis
Muscle

Anatomical

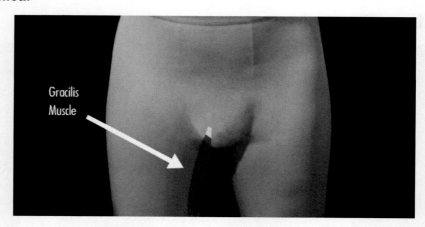

Gracilis
Muscle

The gracilis muscle originates on the pubic tubercle. It is the posterior/medial of the two prominent tendons originating from the pubic tubercles.

Palpation Example

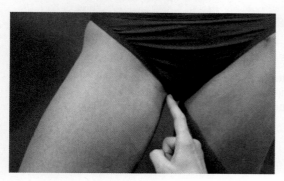

To palpate the gracilis tendon,
1) Place the patient in the supine or supported, standing position.
2) Ask the patient to flex and slightly externally rotate the thigh.
3) Two tendons will become prominent on the superior medial thigh near the pubic tubercle.
4) Locate the tendon that is the more posterior and medial of the two. This tendon is the gracilis tendon.

Greater Trochanter

Skeletal and Anatomical Landmarks

Skeletal

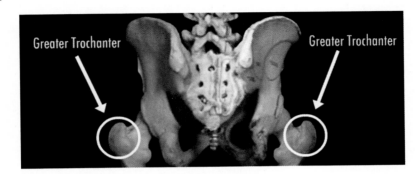

Anatomical

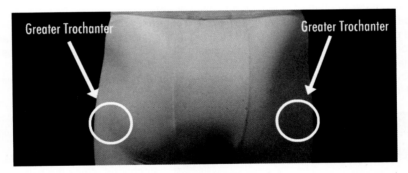

The greater trochanter is the bony prominence located at the widest aspect of the hip.

Palpation Example

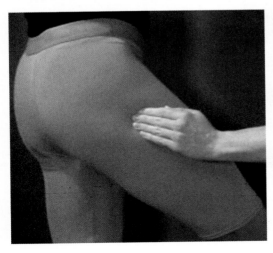

To palpate the greater trochanter,
1) Place the patient in the prone position on the treatment table or standing.
2) To locate the greater trochanter when the patient is standing, ask the patient to flex the hip and internally and externally rotate the femur.
3) Place the palm of your hand on the side of the hip (just posterior to the imaginary seamline of the pants or on the lateral lower edge of the imaginary back pocket) as the patient rotates the leg.
4) The greater trochanter can be felt as it rolls back and forth.
5) Note: If your hand is placed too high, the tensor fascia lata muscle or iliotibial tract will rotate back and forth under your hand, being mistaken for the greater trochanter.

Alternate Method

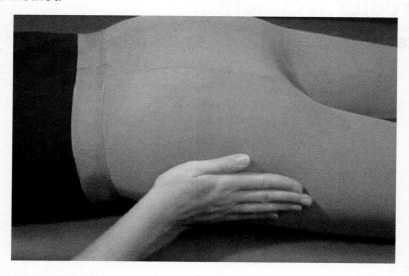

To palpate the greater trochanter when the patient is prone,
1) Ask the patient to flex the knee, then internally and externally rotate the femur.
2) Place the palm of your hand on the side of the hip (just posterior to the imaginary seamline of the pants or on the lateral lower edge of the imaginary back pocket) as the patient rotates the leg.
3) The greater trochanter can be felt as it rotates back and forth.
4) Note: If your hand is placed too high, the tensor fascia lata muscle or iliotibial tract will rotate back and forth under your hand, being mistaken for the greater trochanter.

TIP

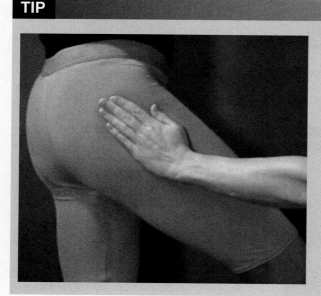

The best to locate the greater trochanter, place the palm of your hand on the side of the hip (just posterior to the imaginary seamline of the pants) as the patient rotates the leg.

◉ Iliac Crest

Skeletal and Anatomical Landmarks

Skeletal

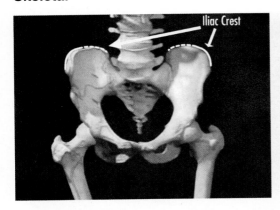

Anatomical

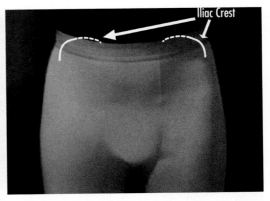

The iliac crest is the superior-most portion of the pelvis. It lies on the lateral aspect of the hip just below the torso. The iliac crest extends from the ASIS to the PSIS.

Palpation Example

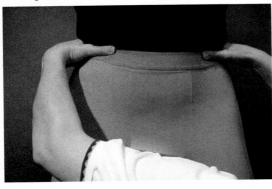

To palpate the iliac crest,
1) Place the patient in either a standing or supine position.
2) With your hands in a pronated position, locate the iliac crests by grasping the patient's sides with the thenar webspace, then pressing into the sides of the body at or just below the waistline to feel the large bony ridge.
3) The thumb and fingers can then be placed on the top of the iliac crest, covering the entire length of the bone.

Alternate Method:

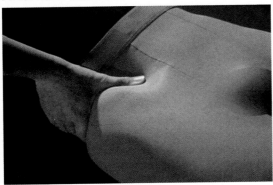

To palpate the iliac crests using an alternate method,
1) Grasp the patient's sides with the thenar webspace just above the waistline, then
2) Slide the hands inferiorly until the bony ridges are felt.
3) Gentle pressure against the body with the thenar webspaces can help locate the iliac crests.

◉ Ischial Tuberosity

Skeletal and Anatomical Landmarks

Skeletal

Anatomical

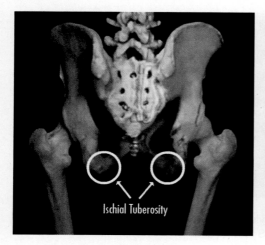

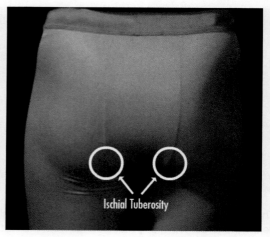

The ischial tuberosity is the inferior aspect of the pelvis. It is often referred to as the butt bone because it is the bone you can feel when you sit.

Palpation Example

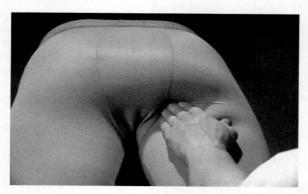

To palpate the ischial tuberosity,
1) Place the patient in either a prone or side-lying position.
2) When the patient is in the prone position, the ischial tuberosity can be located by drawing an imaginary line across the gluteal fold and another line bisecting the buttock medially and laterally.
3) Place two fingers on the gluteal fold line, medial to the line bisecting the buttock, then
4) Press in at a 45 degree angle toward the abdomen.
5) The ischeal tuberosity is felt as a small hard mass under the second finger.

Alternate Method

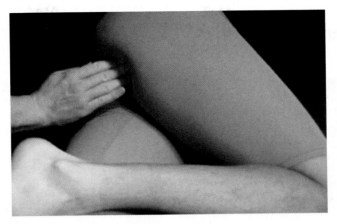

If palpating in the side-lying position,
1) Ask the patient to flex the hip to 90 degrees to make the bone more prominent.
2) Place the palm of your hand on the bottom, medial side of the buttock where the patient would sit on a chair.
3) Press upward toward the head.
4) The ischial tuberosity can be felt as a small hard mass directly in line with the body.

TIP

Imaginary Lines

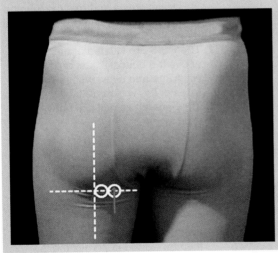

When the patient is in the prone position, the ischial tuberosity can be located by drawing an imaginary line across the gluteal fold and another line bisecting the buttock medially and laterally. The evaluator places the fingers on the gluteal fold line, medial to the line bisecting the buttock, then presses in at a 45 degree angle. The ischial tuberosity is felt as a small hard mass under the second finger.

Posterior Superior Iliac Spine

Skeletal and Anatomical Landmarks

Skeletal

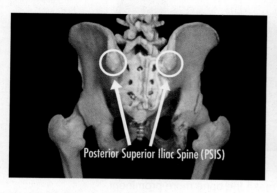

Posterior Superior Iliac Spine (PSIS)

Anatomical

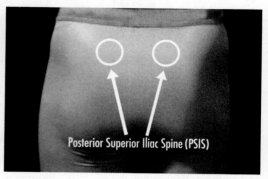

Posterior Superior Iliac Spine (PSIS)

The posterior superior iliac spine (PSIS) is the posterior-most aspect of the iliac bone.

Palpation Example

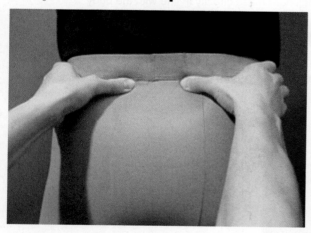

To palpate the posterior superior iliac spine (PSIS) of the patient who is standing,
1) Place your hands on the patient's waist/iliac crests and rest the thumbs down on the body, inferior to the level of the iliac crests.
2) The PSIS are located at the dimples above the buttocks, just below the waist line and a few inches to the sides of the vertebrae.
3) They are felt as ball-like bony prominences.

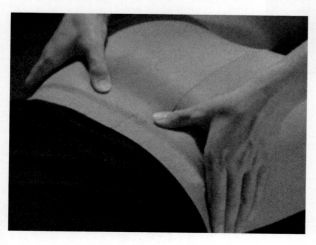

To palpate the posterior superior iliac spine (PSIS) of the patient who is prone,
1) Place your hands on the patient's waist/iliac crest region with your thumbs extended across the low back.
2) The PSIS lie below the waist line, inferior to the level of the iliac crest.
3) They can be felt as small hard protrusions about 2 inches from the midline of the back and 2 inches below the waistline.
4) They are located in the "dimples" of the low back.

⦿ Pubic Tubercles

Skeletal and Anatomical Landmarks

Skeletal   **Anatomical**

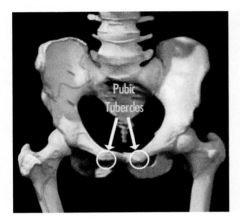 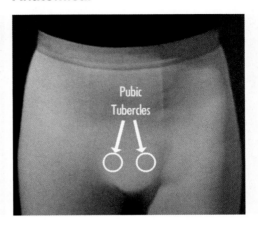

The pubic tubercles are the most prominent anterior bony protrusions in the pubic area.

Palpation Example

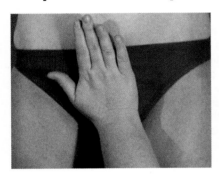

To palpate the pubic tubercles,
1) Place the patient in the supine or standing position.
2) Using the heel of the hand, start around the bikini line.
3) Move inferiorly in a stepwise fashion and press in gently until the bony protrusion is felt.

To palpate the pubic tubercles using an alternate method,
1) Grasp the lateral aspects of the pelvis below the level of the anterior superior iliac spine (ASIS).
2) Move the thumbs toward the pubic tubercles.
3) While visualizing the location of the tubercles, gently press the thumbs against the tubercles.

Self-Palpation:
1) The patient can also perform a self-palpation by locating the most prominent part of the bone for you.

Alternate View - Thumbs   **Self-Palpation**

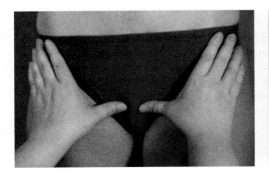 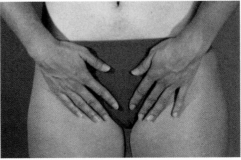

⊙ Rectus Femoris Muscle and Tendon

Skeletal and Anatomical Landmarks

Skeletal

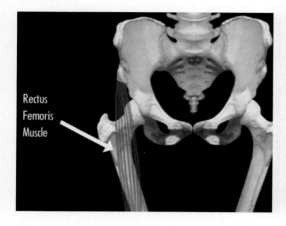

Anatomical

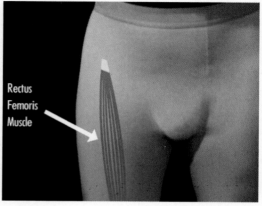

The rectus femoris muscle originates at the anterior inferior iliac spine of the pelvis and joins into the quadriceps tendon before attaching to the patella. It acts as a hip flexor and knee extensor.

Palpation Example

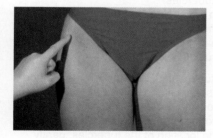

To palpate the rectus femoris muscle,
1) Place the patient in the supine position on the treatment table or ask the patient to stand.
2) If possible, ask the patient to gently contract their muscles in an attempt to flex the hip.
3) Locate the prominent tendons at the anterior crease of the hip, about 2 inches distal to the ASIS.
4) The lateral tendon is the tensor fascia lata tendon; the medial tendon is the sartorius tendon.
5) Palpate between those tendons and move slightly distally (1–2 inches).
6) The rectus femoris tendon can be felt deep in this space.
7) Follow the tendon distally 1–2 inches to palpate the muscle.
8) The muscle then extends down the midthigh to the patella.

TIP

Differentiating the Muscles

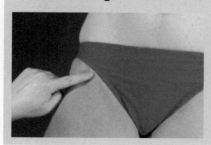

If the patient flexes the hip, the muscles and tendons become more prominent near the ASIS. The lateral tendon is the tensor fascia lata tendon and the medial tendon is the sartorius tendon. The rectus femoris tendon lies deep between the two. The rectus femoris muscle becomes prominent 2–3 inches down the thigh.

● Sacrum

Skeletal and Anatomical Landmarks

Skeletal   **Anatomical**

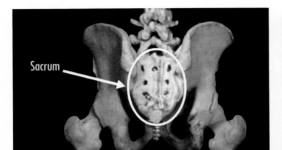

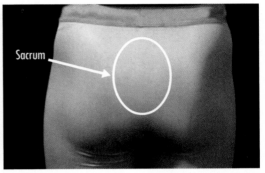

The sacrum is inferior to the lumbar spine and superior to the coccyx. The superior aspect of the sacrum lies at the level of the PSIS.

Palpation Example

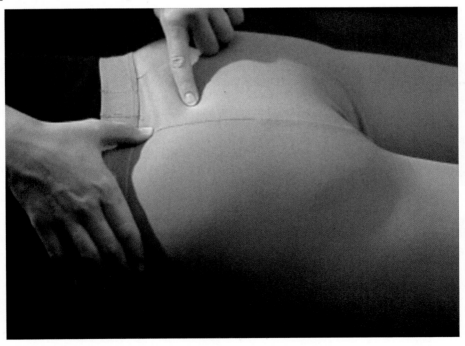

To palpate the sacrum,
1) Place the patient in the prone position on the treatment table.
2) Locate the PSIS, then
3) Move medially to the vertebral column.
4) The sacrum starts at this level and extends approximately 4 to 5 inches (1–1½ hand widths) distally, just beyond the start of the gluteal crease.

⦿ Sartorius Muscle

Skeletal and Anatomical Landmarks

Skeletal   **Anatomical**

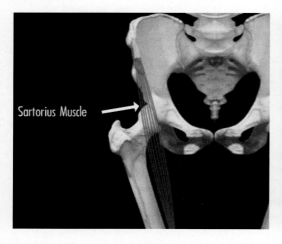

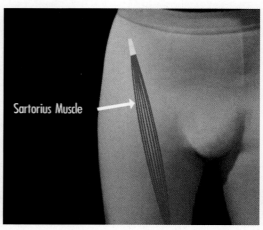

The sartorius muscle is a long ribbonlike muscle that originates at the ASIS, crosses the anterior thigh, and inserts at the pes anserine.

Palpation Example

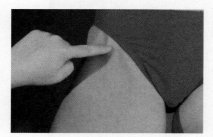

To palpate the sartorius muscle and its proximal tendon,
1) Place the patient in the supine position on the treatment table.
2) If possible, ask the patient to slightly flex and externally rotate the hip.
3) Locate the tendons that become very prominent at the anterior crease of the hip, just distal to the ASIS.
4) The sartorius tendon is the more medial of the two tendons.
5) It lies near the midline of the anterior hip and can be palpated for several inches distally as it becomes the muscle.

TIP

Differentiating the Muscles

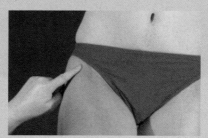

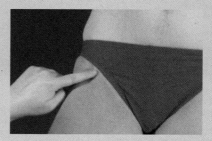

To differentiate the tendons at the anterior hip, ask the patient to flex the hip and slightly externally rotate the thigh. Three tendons/muscles can be felt. The more prominent medial tendon is the sartorius, the lateral tendon is that of tensor fascia lata, and tendon that lies between the two and slightly more distally is the rectus femoris.

◉ Sciatic Nerve

Skeletal and Anatomical Landmarks

Skeletal   **Anatomical**

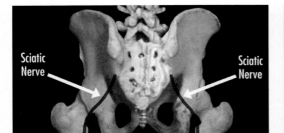
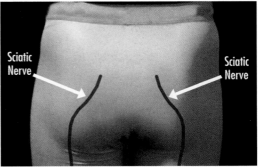

The sciatic nerve lies midway between the greater trochanter and the ischial tuberosity.

Palpation Example

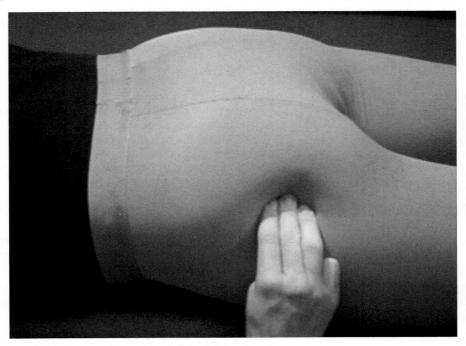

To palpate the sciatic nerve,
1) Place the patient in the prone position on the treatment table.
2) Locate the greater trochanter, then
3) Move a few inches onto the buttocks toward the ischial tuberosity.
4) Locate the distinct groove posterior and medial to the greater trochanter.
5) The sciatic nerve lies deep in this groove, half way between the greater trochanter and the ischial tuberosity.
6) Palpate straight into the groove using 2 or 3 fingers.

● Tensor Fascia Lata Muscle

Skeletal and Anatomical Landmarks

Skeletal   **Anatomical**

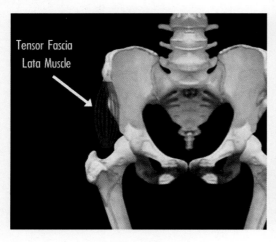
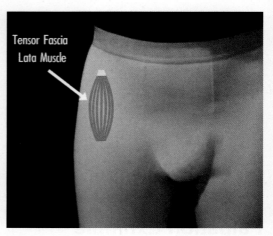

The tensor fascia lata muscle originates at the ASIS and inserts into the iliotibial (IT) band. The IT band then inserts at Gerdy tubercle. The TFL muscle is primarily a hip abductor, but it also has accessory motions and stabilizing functions at both the hip and the knee.

Palpation Example

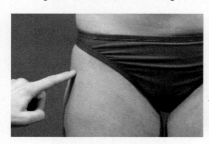

To palpate the TFL muscle,
1) Place the patient in the supine position on the treatment table or in a standing position.
2) If possible, ask the patient to slightly flex and internally and externally rotate the hip.
3) Locate the tendons that become very prominent at the anterior crease of the hip, just distal to the ASIS.
4) The TFL tendon is the more lateral of the two tendons and is felt best when the hip is internally rotated and slightly flexed and abducted.
5) Move distally along the tendon 2–3 inches to the TFL muscle.
6) It lies distal to the ASIS about 45 degrees between the frontal and sagittal planes and can be palpated for a few inches.

TIP

Differentiating the Muscles

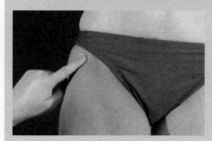

To differentiate the tendons at the anterior hip, ask the patient to flex the hip and slightly externally and internally rotate the thigh. Three tendons/muscles can be felt. The lateral tendon is the TFL, the medial tendon is that of sartorius, and the tendon that lies between the two and slightly more distally is the rectus femoris.

● Adductor Tubercle

Skeletal and Anatomical Landmarks

Skeletal

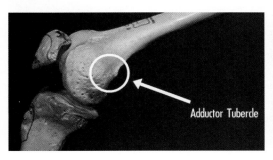

Adductor Tubercle

Anatomical

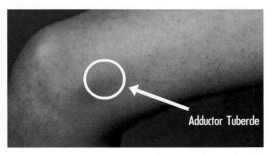

Adductor Tubercle

The adductor tubercle is located on the posterior medial aspect of the medial epicondyle.

Palpation Example

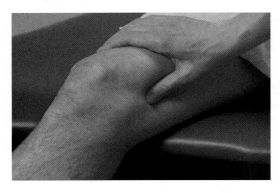

To palpate the adductor tubercle,
1) Place the patient in a seated position at the end of the treatment table or supine on the treatment table. Stand in front of the seated patient or to the side of the supine patient.
2) Starting on the distal third of the medial thigh (at the imaginary seamline of the pants), press in and move distally toward the medial epicondyle of the knee.
3) You will pass through a softer indented area in the muscle just superior to the knee before running into a larger bony ridge. The adductor tubercle is the posterior medial aspect of that bony ridge. It is tender to palpate.

TIP

Seamline of Pants

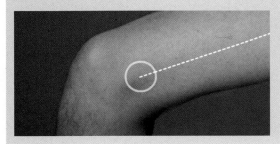

The adductor tubercle is located on the medial distal thigh along the imaginary seamline of the pants.

◉ Biceps Femoris Tendon

Skeletal and Anatomical Landmarks

Skeletal

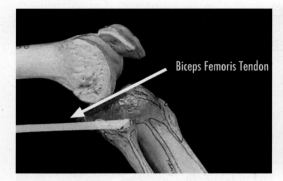

Biceps Femoris Tendon

Anatomical

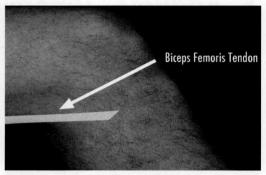

Biceps Femoris Tendon

The biceps femoris is the lateral-most hamstring muscle. Its tendon crosses the knee at the posterior lateral aspect of the knee.

Palpation Example

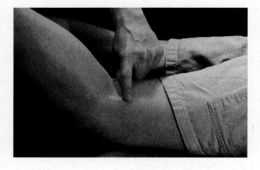

To palpate the biceps femoris tendon,
1) Place the patient in a seated position at the end of the treatment table or prone on the treatment table. Stand to the side of the prone patient or facing a seated patient.
2) Ask the patient to flex the knee against resistance.
3) Locate the prominent tendon that appears as a thick "cord" on the lateral aspect of the posterior knee.
4) The tendon can be palpated with the fingers or by gently pinching the tendon between the thumb and fingers.

Alternate Method

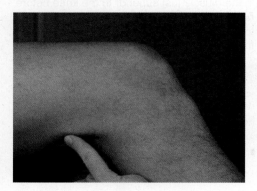

The tendon can also be palpated while the patient is in the seated position.

● Common Peroneal Nerve

Skeletal and Anatomical Landmarks

Skeletal   **Anatomical**

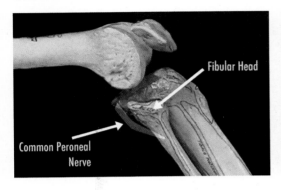

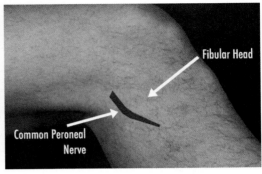

The common peroneal nerve wraps around behind the fibular head.

Palpation Example

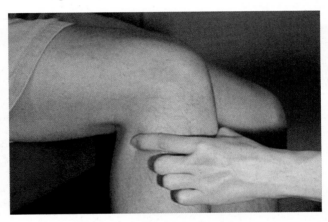

To palpate the common peroneal nerve,
1) Place the patient in a seated position at the end of the treatment table.
2) Locate the fibular head, then move distally to the lateral portion of the "neck" of the fibula.
3) The nerve can be felt as a spongier band that runs anteriorly around the bone.
4) Strumming back and forth across the nerve in an anterior-superior to posterior-inferior pattern may help locate the nerve.
5) The nerve should be palpated gently to prevent injuring it.

● Fibular Head

Skeletal and Anatomical Landmarks

Skeletal   **Anatomical**

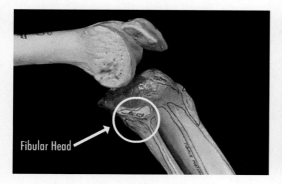

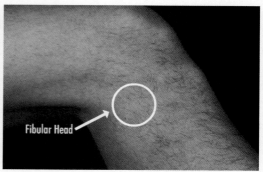

The fibular head is located on the lateral aspect of the leg just below the joint line of the knee. It is at the approximate level of the tibial tubercle.

Palpation Example

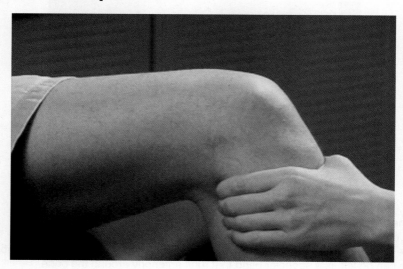

To palpate the head of the fibula,
1) Place the patient in a seated position at the end of the treatment table. Sit on a stool facing the patient. Use your left hand for the patient's right knee or your right hand for the patient's left knee.
2) With your index finger at the joint line and your thenar webspace on the patellar tendon, grip the patient's leg.
3) Wrap your fingers around the lateral aspect of the leg.
4) In this position, your middle and/or ring fingers should be gripping the posterior and lateral aspects of the fibular head, which can be felt as a bony prominence.
5) Pull your fingers back to the lateral-most aspect of the bony prominence to palpate the main portion of the fibular head.
6) The landmark can be verified by asking the patient to medially and laterally rotate the lower leg as you continue to palpate. The fibular head will be felt rotating back and forth under your finger.

Alternate Method

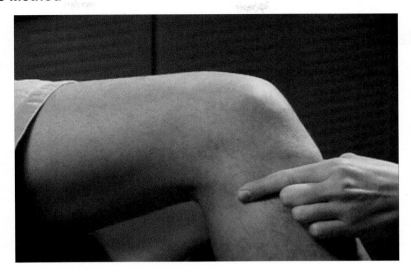

To palpate the head of the fibula using an alternate method,
1) Place the patient in a seated position at the end of the treatment table. Sit on a stool facing the patient. Use your left hand for the patient's right knee or your right hand for the patient's left knee.
2) Locate the joint line of the knee then move laterally along the joint line with your index finger to the lateral collateral ligament.
3) From this point, move one or two finger widths distally where you will feel a larger bony prominence.
4) To feel the most prominent portion of the fibular head, you may have to move one or two finger widths posteriorly.

⦿ Gerdy's Tubercle

Skeletal and Anatomical Landmarks

Skeletal

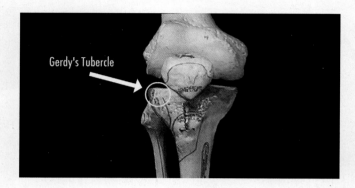

Anatomical

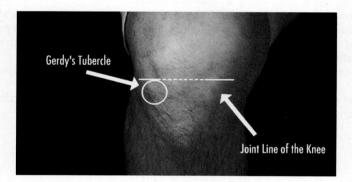

Gerdy's tubercle is located on the anterior lateral border of the tibia just distal to the joint line of the knee. It serves as the attachment site for the iliotibial band.

Palpation Example

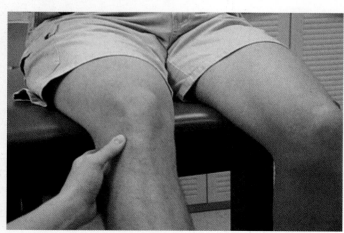

To palpate Gerdy's tubercle,
1) Place the patient in a seated position at the end of the treatment table.
2) Locate the joint line of the knee just lateral to the patellar tendon, then
3) Move distally onto the tibia.
4) Gerdy's tubercle is the large bony protrusion that is felt approximately 1–2 finger widths below the joint line.

● Iliotibial Tract

Skeletal and Anatomical Landmarks

Skeletal

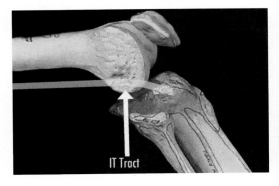

Anatomical

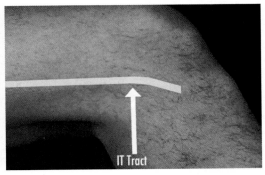

The iliotibial (IT) tract (often referred to as the IT band) crosses the lateral knee joint near the lateral epicondyle and inserts on Gerdy's tubercle.

Palpation Example

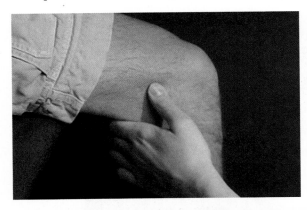

To palpate the IT tract,
1) Place the patient in a seated position at the end of the treatment table.
2) Locate the lateral epicondyle, then
3) Move proximally about one inch.
4) The IT tract can be felt as a tighter band when you rub back and forth across it.
5) To verify the palpation of the IT tract, ask the patient to extend and flex the knee. The IT tract should roll back and forth under your finger.

TIP

Flex and Extend the Knee
To verify the palpation of the IT tract, ask the patient to extend and flex the knee. The IT tract should roll back and forth under your finger, moving anteriorly as the patient extends the knee and posteriorly as the patient flexes the knee.

⊙ Infrapatellar Bursa

Skeletal and Anatomical Landmarks

Skeletal

Anatomical

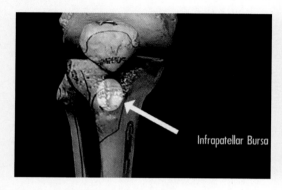

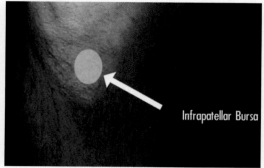

The infrapatellar bursae lie inferior to the patella. One bursa lies deep to the distal patellar tendon, while the other lies superficial to the tendon.

Palpation Example

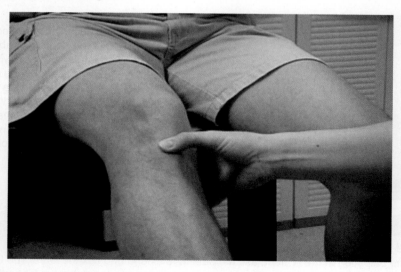

To palpate the infrapatellar bursa,
1) Place the patient in a seated position at the end of the treatment table.
2) Palpate the area along the patellar tendon.
3) The bursa may not be palpable unless inflamed.

Joint Line of the Knee

Skeletal and Anatomical Landmarks

Skeletal

Anatomical

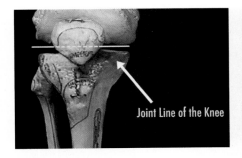

Joint Line of the Knee

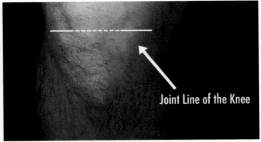

Joint Line of the Knee

The joint line of the knee is the junction of the femur and the tibia.

Palpation Example

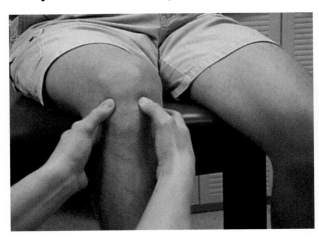

To palpate the joint line of the knee,
1) It is best to have the patient seated at the end of the treatment table with the knee flexed to 90 degrees.
2) Locate the joint line by grasping the tibia with both hands and placing the thumbs to the sides of the patellar tendon.
3) Move the thumbs up and down along the knee until the indentations are felt.
4) The indentations are the anterior portion of the joint line.

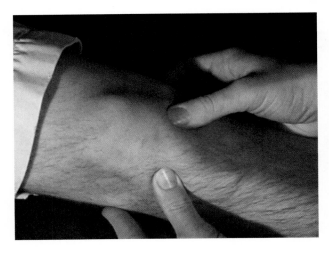

The joint line of the knee can also be palpated while the knee is fully extended. To palpate the joint line from this position,
1) Ensure the quadriceps muscles are relaxed, then
2) Locate the distal border of the patella.
3) The joint line lies at this approximate level and is best palpated by moving the thumbs slightly medially and laterally from the patella then feeling for a slight gap between the femur and tibia.

◉ Lateral Collateral Ligament (Knee)

Skeletal and Anatomical Landmarks

Skeletal

Anatomical

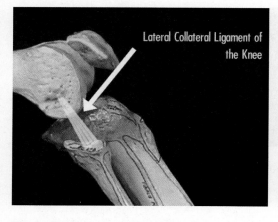

Lateral Collateral Ligament of the Knee

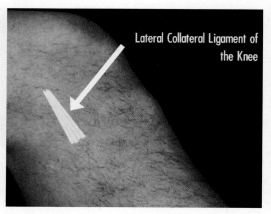

Lateral Collateral Ligament of the Knee

The lateral collateral ligament is a narrow ligament that extends from the lateral epicondyle of the femur to the fibular head.

Palpation Example

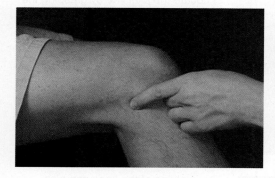

To palpate the lateral collateral ligament of the knee,
1) Place the patient in a seated position at the end of the treatment table.
2) Locate the lateral joint line of the knee, then
3) Move along the joint line to the midpoint of the lateral knee.
4) The ligament is similar to a large rubber band that extends across the joint line. It can be felt by moving the finger back and forth across it.

TIP

Externally Rotate the Thigh

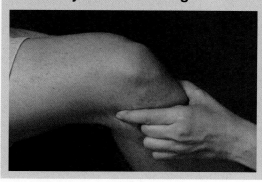

The ligament becomes more prominent when the knee remains flexed and the thigh is externally rotated.

Lateral Epicondyle of the Knee

Skeletal and Anatomical Landmarks

Skeletal   **Anatomical**

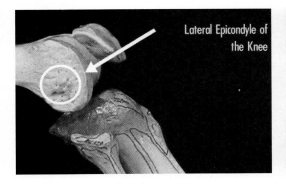

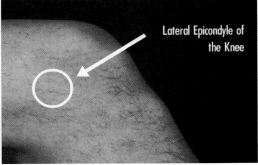

The lateral epicondyle of the knee is the lateral-most bony prominence of the knee, just above the joint line.

Palpation Example

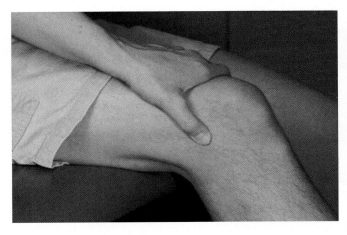

To palpate the lateral epicondyle of the knee,
1) Place the patient in a seated position at the end of the treatment table.
2) Locate the lateral-most bony prominence of the knee, just above the joint line.
3) The epicondyle can often be preliminarily located with the naked eye or by grasping the distal thigh and moving toward the joint line of the knee until the most prominent point is felt.

◉ Medial Collateral Ligament of the Knee

Skeletal and Anatomical Landmarks

Skeletal   **Anatomical**

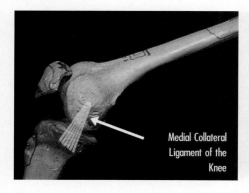

Medial Collateral
Ligament of the
Knee

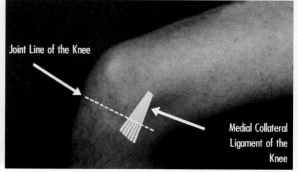

Joint Line of the Knee

Medial Collateral
Ligament of the
Knee

The medial collateral ligament of the knee is located slightly posterior to the center of the medial joint line. It attaches proximally on the medial femoral condyle, distal to the adductor tubercle, and distally to the medial tibial condyle.

Palpation Example

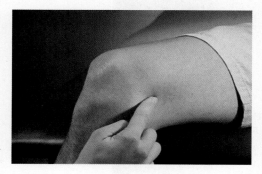

To palpate the medial collateral ligament of the knee,
1) Place the patient in a seated position at the end of the treatment table.
2) Locate the medial joint line of the knee, then
3) Move along the joint line to the midpoint of the medial knee.
4) The ligament is similar to a large rubber band that extends across the joint line.
5) It can be felt by moving the finger back and forth across it.

TIP

Rotate Leg

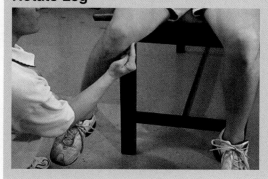

The ligament becomes more prominent when the knee remains flexed and the thigh is internally rotated.

◉ Medial Epicondyle of the Knee

Skeletal and Anatomical Landmarks

Skeletal

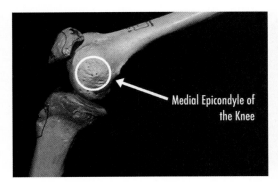

Anatomical

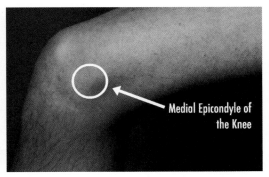

The medial epicondyle of the knee is the medial-most bony prominence on the distal femur. It serves as the attachment site for the medial/tibial collateral ligament.

Palpation Example

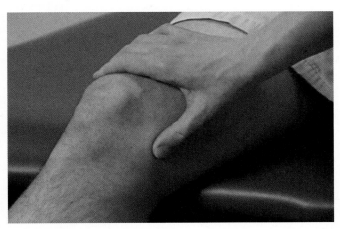

To palpate the medial epicondyle of the knee,
1) Place the patient in a seated position at the end of the treatment table.
2) Locate the medial-most bony prominence of the knee, just above the joint line.
3) The epicondyle can often be preliminarily located with the naked eye or by grasping the distal thigh and moving toward the joint line of the knee until the most prominent point is felt on the medial knee.

● Patella

Skeletal and Anatomical Landmarks

Skeletal   **Anatomical**

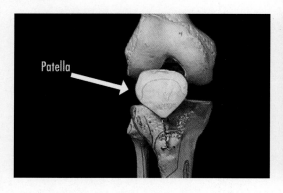
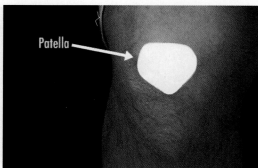

The patella is the bone commonly referred to as the kneecap.

Palpation Example

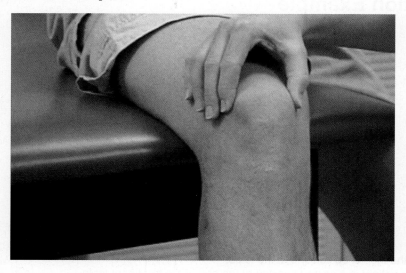

To palpate the patella,
1) Place the patient in a seated position at the end of the treatment table or in a long sit position on the treatment table.
2) Locate the bone that is commonly referred to as the kneecap (the patella) on the front of the knee.
3) Palpate all aspects of the patella including the base (superior portion), the apex (inferior, angular portion), the medial and lateral edges, and the anterior surface.

⊙ Patellar Ligament

Skeletal and Anatomical Landmarks

Skeletal

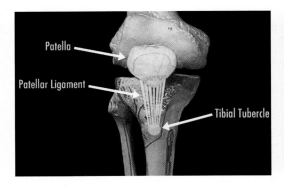

Anatomical

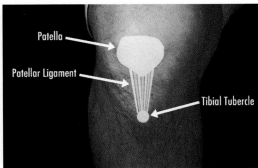

The patellar tendon (often referred to as the patellar ligament) attaches proximally to the patella and distally to the tibial tubercle.

Palpation Example

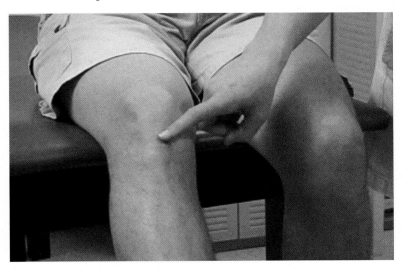

To palpate the patellar tendon (or patellar ligament),
1) Place the patient in a seated position at the end of the treatment table or in a long sit position on the treatment table.
2) Locate the inferior border of the patella where the tendon originates.
3) Follow the thick tendon distally to its distal attachment on the tibial tubercle.

◉ Pes Anserine

Skeletal and Anatomical Landmarks

Skeletal

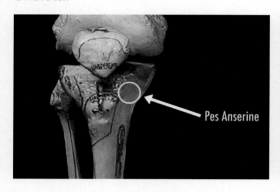

Anatomical

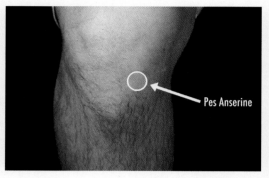

The pes anserine is located on the anterior medial aspect of the superior tibia, medial to the patellar tendon. It serves as the attachment site for the sartorius, gracilis, and semitendinosus tendons.

Palpation Example

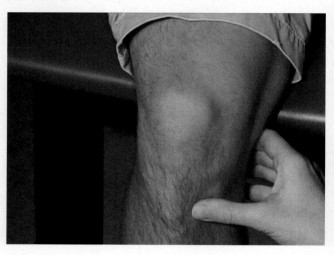

To palpate the pes anserine,
1) Place the patient in a seated position at the end of the treatment table.
2) Locate the medial joint line, then
3) Move distally, past the tibial plateau to the flatter portion of the bone that is about 2 inches below the joint line.
4) This area is the pes anserine.

◉ Pes Anserine Bursa

Skeletal and Anatomical Landmarks

Skeletal   **Anatomical**

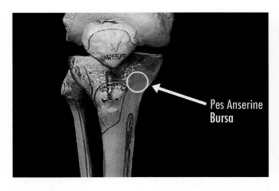   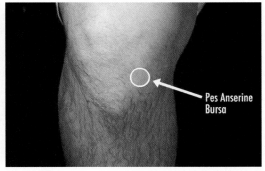

The pes anserine bursa is located on the anterior medial aspect of the superior tibia, medial to the patellar tendon. It covers the pes anserine and serves as a cushion between the bone and the sartorius, gracilis, and semitendinosus tendons.

Palpation Example

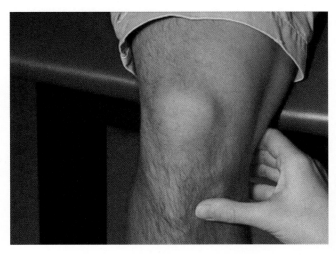

To palpate the pes anserine bursa,
1) Place the patient in a seated position at the end of the treatment table.
2) Locate the medial joint line, then
3) Move distally, past the tibial plateau to the flatter portion of the bone that is about 2 inches below the joint line.
4) This area is the pes anserine and contains the pes anserine bursa.
5) The bursa is not palpable unless inflamed.

◉ Popliteal Fossa

Skeletal and Anatomical Landmarks

Skeletal	Anatomical

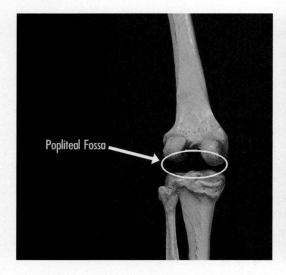
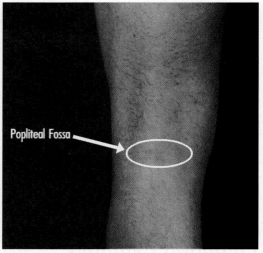

The popliteal fossa is the large divot between the hamstring tendons at the joint crease on the posterior aspect of the knee.

Palpation Example

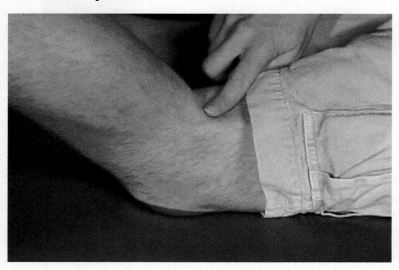

To best visualize and palpate the popliteal fossa,
1) Place the patient in the prone position on the treatment table.
2) Ask the patient to attempt to flex the knee against slight resistance.
3) Locate the large divot that appears between the medial and lateral hamstring tendons.
4) This divot is the popliteal fossa.

● Prepatellar Bursa

Skeletal and Anatomical Landmarks

Skeletal

Anatomical

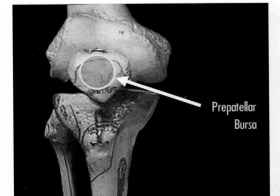

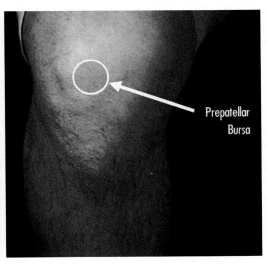

The prepatellar bursa lies on the anterior surface of the patella.

Palpation Example

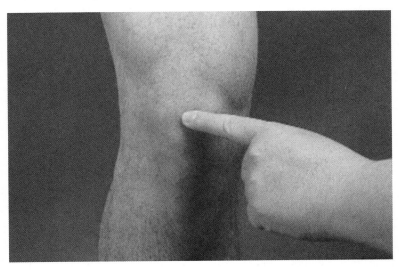

To palpate the prepatellar bursa,
1) Place the patient in a seated position at the end of the treatment table or in a long sit position on the treatment table.
2) Locate the patella and palpate its anterior surface.
3) The bursa lies on the anterior surface but may not be palpable unless it is inflamed.

◉ Quadriceps Tendon

Skeletal and Anatomical Landmarks

Skeletal

Anatomical

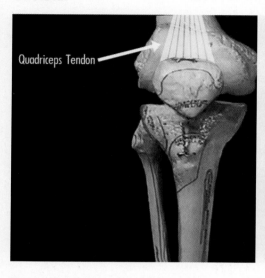
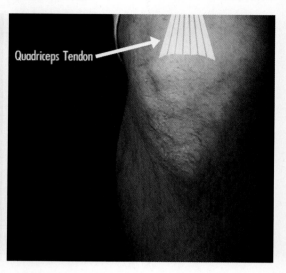

The quadriceps tendon attaches the quadriceps muscles to the patella.

Palpation Example

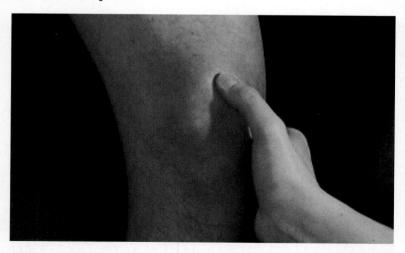

To palpate the quadriceps tendon,
1) Place the patient in a seated position at the end of the treatment table or in a long sit position on the treatment table.
2) The quadriceps tendon attaches the quadriceps muscles to the patella.
3) Locate the tendon just proximal to the patella.
4) Using your fingers or thumb, palpate the tendon's full length 1–2 inches above the patella as well as its attachment site along the superior border of the patella.
5) Asking the patient to contract the quadriceps muscles will make the tendon become more prominent.

● Semimembranosus Tendon

Skeletal and Anatomical Landmarks

Skeletal

Anatomical

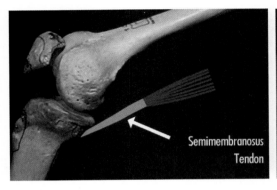 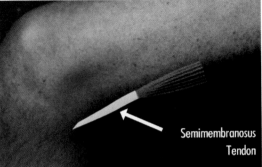

The semimembranosus muscle is the medial-most hamstring muscle. It originates on the ischial tuberosity and inserts on the posterior medial tibia. Its tendon crosses the knee just medial to the semitendinosus tendon.

Palpation Example

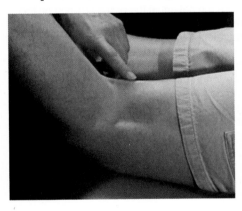

To palpate the semimembranosus tendon,
1) Place the patient in the prone position on the treatment table or seated at the end of the treatment table.
2) Ask the patient to flex the knee against slight resistance.
3) The tendon that becomes the most visible and palpable as a thick "cord" on the medial aspect of the posterior knee is the semitendinosus tendon.
4) Locate that tendon, then move about one finger width medially to the second, less visible and palpable tendon.
5) That second tendon is the semimembranosus tendon.
6) It can be palpated for several inches.

Alternate View

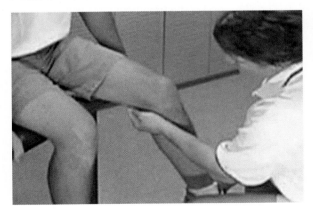

The patient can also be seated at the end of the treatment table with the knee flexed 90 degrees.
1) In this position, the evaluator reaches around the posterior medial aspect of the knee and locates the cord-like structure just proximal to the joint line.
2) The most prominent tendon is the semitendinosus tendon.
3) Move about one finger width medially to the second, less visible and palpable tendon.
5) That second tendon is the semimembranosus tendon.

● Semitendinosus Tendon

Skeletal and Anatomical Landmarks

Skeletal   **Anatomical**

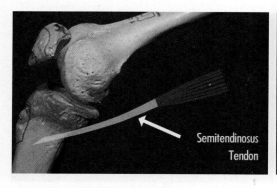

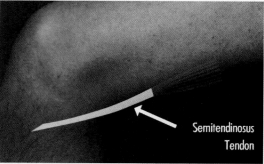

The semitendinosus tendon is the lateral of the two hamstring tendons on the posterior medial aspect of the knee. It attaches to the pes anserine.

Palpation Example

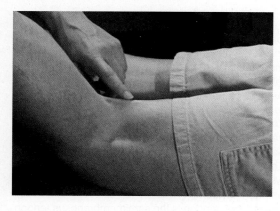

To palpate the semitendinosus tendon,
1) Place the patient in the prone position on the treatment table or seated at the end of the treatment table.
2) Ask the patient to flex the knee against slight resistance.
3) The tendon that becomes the most visible and palpable as a thick "cord" on the medial aspect of the posterior knee is the semitendinosus tendon.
4) It can be palpated for several inches.

Alternate View

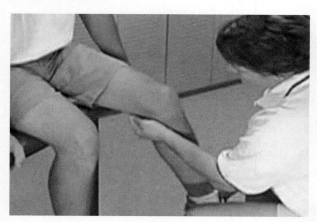

The patient can also be seated at the end of the treatment table with the knee flexed 90 degrees.
1) In this position, the evaluator reaches around the posterior medial aspect of the knee and locates the cordlike structure just proximal to the joint line.
2) The most prominent tendon is the semitendinosus tendon.

◉ Suprapatellar Bursa

Skeletal and Anatomical Landmarks

Skeletal

Anatomical

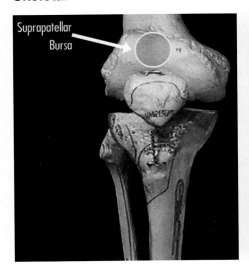 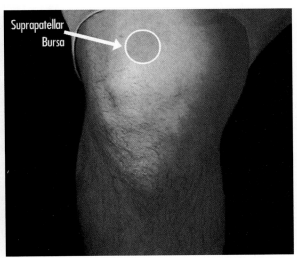

The suprapatellar bursa lies between the distal femur and the quadriceps tendon.

Palpation Example

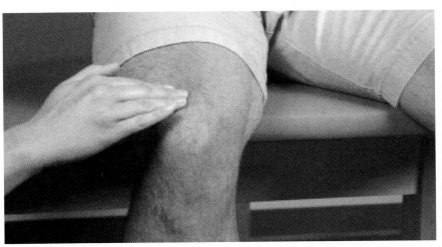

To palpate the suprapatellar bursa,
1) Place the patient in a seated position at the end of the treatment table.
2) Palpate along the lateral edges of the quadriceps tendon as well as pressing on the tendon itself for an indirect palpation.
3) The bursa may not be easily distinguishable unless it is inflamed.

◉ Tibial Plateau

Skeletal and Anatomical Landmarks

Skeletal   **Anatomical**

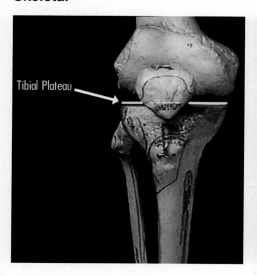
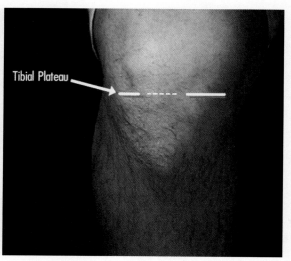

The tibial plateau is the superior-most aspect of the tibia on which the menisci rest.

Palpation Example

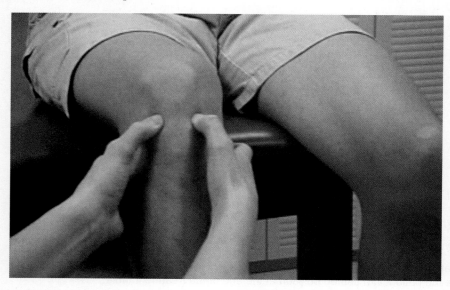

To palpate the tibial plateau,
1) Place the patient in a seated position at the end of the treatment table.
2) Locate the joint line of the knee.
3) With the thumbs in the anterior joint space, press inferiorly on the tibia.
4) The thumbs will be resting on the anterior border of the tibial plateau.

◉ Tibial Tubercle

Skeletal and Anatomical Landmarks

Skeletal

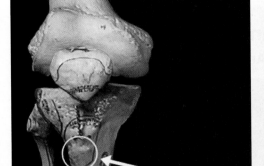

Anatomical

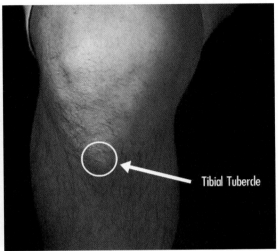

Tibial Tubercle

Tibial Tubercle

The tibial tubercle is a bony prominence on the superior anterior tibia to which the patellar tendon attaches.

Palpation Example

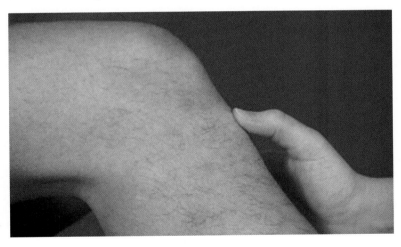

To palpate the tibial tubercle (tuberosity),
1) Place the patient in a seated position at the end of the treatment table.
2) Locate the large bony prominence (the tibial tubercle) on the superior anterior aspect of the tibia, 2–3 finger widths below the joint line of the knee.
3) The tuberosity serves as the distal attachment site for the patellar tendon and can be palpated by locating the patellar tendon (ligament) then moving distally until the tendon meets the tibia.

◉ Achilles Tendon

Skeletal and Anatomical Landmarks

Skeletal

Anatomical

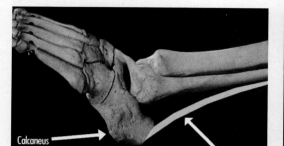

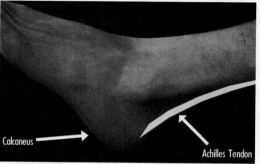

The Achilles tendon is the common tendon for the gastrocnemius and soleus muscles. It runs from the distal calf to its insertion on the posterior calcaneus.

Palpation Example

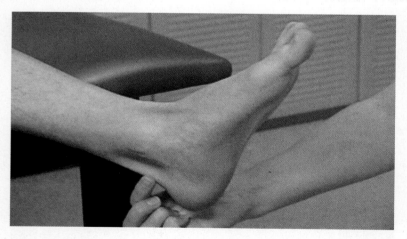

To palpate the Achilles tendon,
1) Place the patient either prone or in a long sit position on the treatment table or standing, facing away from the evaluator.
2) Locate the large ropelike tendon at the back of the lower leg and ankle.
3) Pinch the tendon between the thumb and fingers or press with the fingers along the full length of the tendon.
4) The tendon can be palpated from the gastrocnemius muscle to the calcaneus.
5) Palpate the medial edge, lateral edge, and center of the tendon.

◉ Anterior Talofibular Ligament

Skeletal and Anatomical Landmarks

Skeletal   **Anatomical**

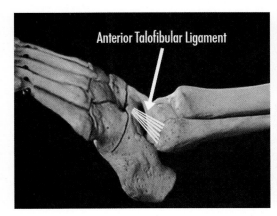 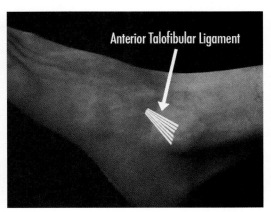

The anterior talofibular ligament lies in the sinus tarsi. It attaches the distal fibula to the anterior talus.

Palpation Example

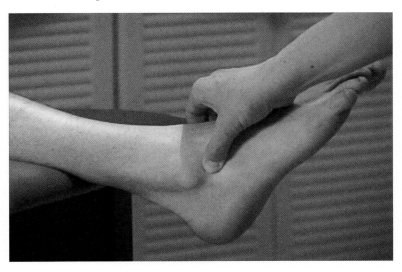

To palpate the anterior talofibular ligament,
1) Place the patient in a seated position at the end of the treatment table or in a long sit position on the treatment table.
2) Locate the lateral malleolus, then move anteriorly into the sinus tarsi.
3) The ligament can be felt as a short, thin band deep in the sinus tarsi along the anterior border of the lateral malleolus.
4) Pressure in an anterior-posterior motion may be needed to locate the ligament.

Anterior Tibiofibular Ligament

Skeletal and Anatomical Landmarks

Skeletal

Anatomical

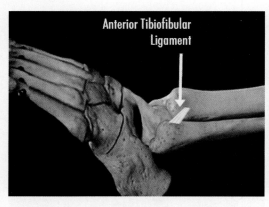

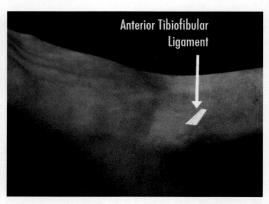

The anterior tibiofibular ligament is located superior to the lateral malleolus and anterior to the shaft of the fibula.

Palpation Example

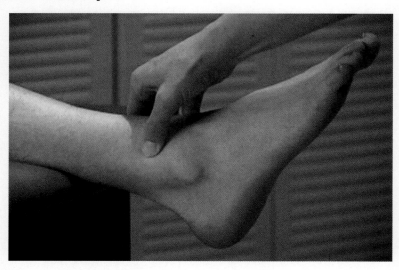

To palpate the anterior tibiofibular ligament,
1) Place the patient in a seated position at the end of the treatment table or in a long sit position on the treatment table.
2) Locate the lateral malleolus then move 2–3 finger widths proximally along the fibular shaft and anteriorly to the edge of the fibula.
3) Palpate with a single digit or pinch the front and back of the fibula between the thumb and fingers and move in a short superior-inferior motion along the shaft.
4) The ligament may not be distinguishable but pain in the area may be experienced if the ligament is injured.

◉ Base of the 5th Metatarsal

Skeletal and Anatomical Landmarks

Skeletal

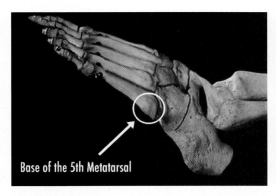

Base of the 5th Metatarsal

Anatomical

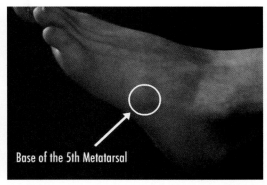

Base of the 5th Metatarsal

The base of the 5th metatarsal is the large protrusion on the lateral aspect of the foot about halfway between the metatarsal head and the calcaneus.

Palpation Example

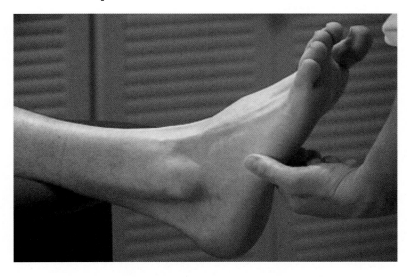

To palpate the base of the 5th metatarsal (also called the styloid process),
1) Place the patient in a seated position at the end of the treatment table or in a long sit position on the treatment table.
2) Locate the head of the 5th metatarsal, then slide proximally on the lateral-most aspect of the foot.
3) The base of the 5th metatarsal can be felt as a large protrusion approximately halfway up the foot.
4) There will also be a larger divot just proximal to the base of the 5th metatarsal, alerting you that you have passed the bone.
5) The bone can be palpated with a single digit or by gently pinching the bone between the thumb and fingers.

⊙ Calcaneofibular Ligament

Skeletal and Anatomical Landmarks

Skeletal   **Anatomical**

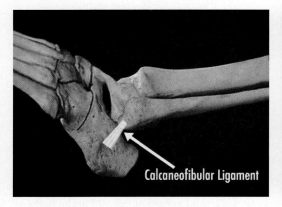 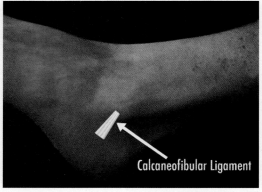

The calcaneofibular ligament is located just inferior to the lateral malleolus. It connects the distal tip of the malleolus to the calcaneus.

Palpation Example

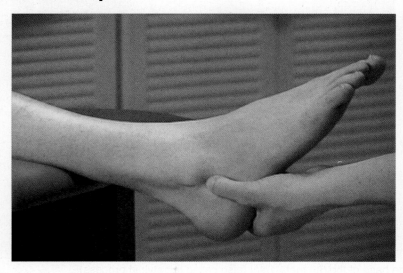

To palpate the calcaneofibular ligament,
1) Place the patient in a seated or long sit position on the treatment table.
2) Locate the lateral malleolus then move inferiorly, just off the malleolus.
3) The calcaneofibular ligament is felt as a short, narrow band.
4) Moving the finger anteriorly and posteriorly over the tendon will help locate the tendon.

◉ Cuboid

Skeletal and Anatomical Landmarks

Skeletal   **Anatomical**

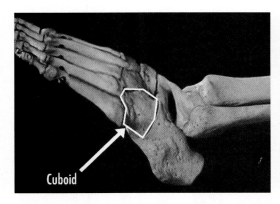

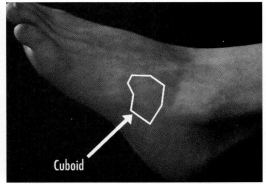

The cuboid is a larger, flat bone located proximal to the base of the 5th metatarsal and lateral to the 3rd cuneiform.

Palpation Example

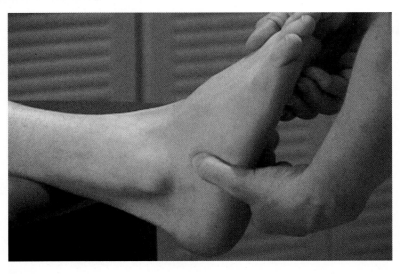

To palpate the cuboid,
1) Place the patient in a seated or long sit position on the treatment table.
2) Locate the base of the 5th metatarsal, then move proximally one finger width into the divot behind the base of the 5th metatarsal.
3) The cuboid lies in this divot and extends about 2 finger widths medially onto the top of the foot.

⊙ Cuneiforms

Skeletal and Anatomical Landmarks

Skeletal	Anatomical

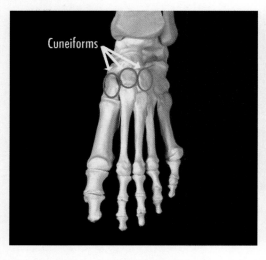 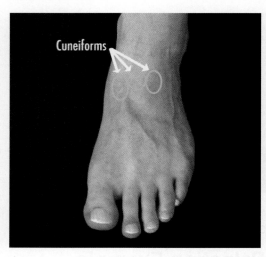

The cuneiforms lie distal to the navicular and proximal to the 1st, 2nd, and 3rd metatarsals.

Palpation Example

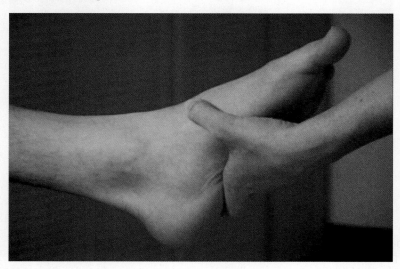

To palpate the cuneiforms,
1) Place the patient in a seated or long sit position on the treatment table.
2) Locate the navicular tubercle, then move distally one finger width.
3) This bone is the 1st cuneiform.
4) The 2nd and 3rd cuneiforms lie in a row lateral to 1st and extend to the midline of the foot.

Deltoid Ligament

Skeletal and Anatomical Landmarks

Skeletal   **Anatomical**

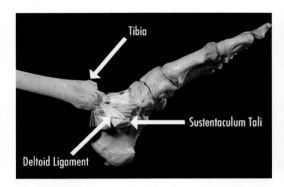

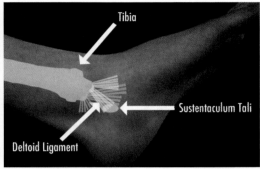

The deltoid ligament is made up of four separate ligaments. These individual ligaments connect the distal tibia to the anterior talus, the navicular, the calcaneus, and the posterior talus to form a large fan-shaped structure.

Palpation Example

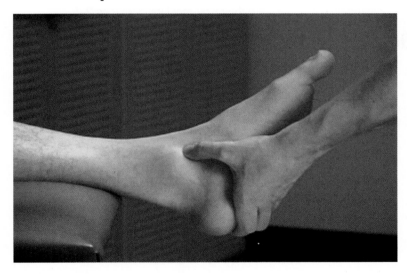

To palpate the deltoid ligament,
1) Place the patient in a seated or long sit position on the treatment table.
2) Locate the medial malleolus, then move anteriorly just off the bone into a groove. The deltoid ligament crosses this groove and fans the full distal aspect of the malleolus.
3) Following the outline of the malleolus, palpate in the groove to the posterior portion of the malleolus, ensuring all portions of the deltoid ligament are palpated.

⊙ Distal Interphalangeal Joints (Foot)

Skeletal and Anatomical Landmarks

Skeletal   **Anatomical**

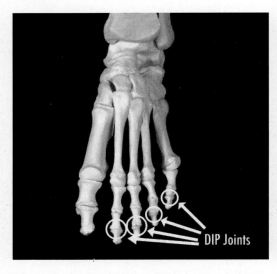

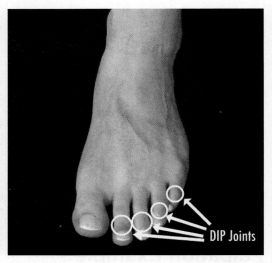

The distal interphalangeal (DIP) joints are the distal-most joints of toes 2–5.

Palpation Example

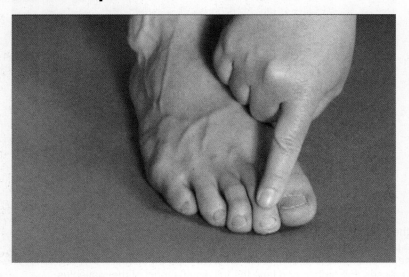

To palpate the DIP joints of the foot,
1) Place the patient in a seated or long sit position on the treatment table with the toes extended.
2) Locate the most distal joint on toes 2–5.
3) The joints can be palpated with a single digit or by pinching the joint gently between the finger and thumb.
4) The joints should be palpated on all sides.

● Dome of the Talus

Skeletal and Anatomical Landmarks

Skeletal

Anatomical

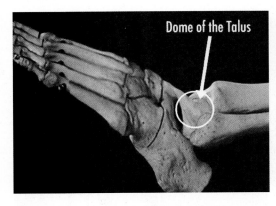

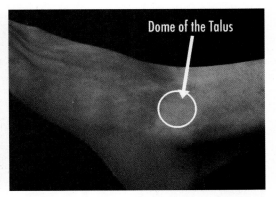

The dome of the talus is located in the anterior sinus tarsi.

Palpation Example

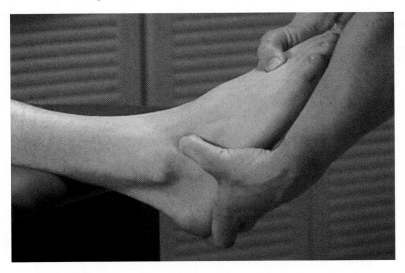

To palpate the dome of the talus,
1) Place the patient in a seated or long sit position on the treatment table.
2) Locate the sinus tarsi and place your thumb in the sinus tarsi.
3) With the thumb in place, passively invert the ankle with the opposite hand.
4) A bone will become prominent under the thumb in the sinus tarsi. This bone is the dome of the talus.

◉ Dorsal Pedal Pulse

Skeletal and Anatomical Landmarks

Skeletal   **Anatomical**

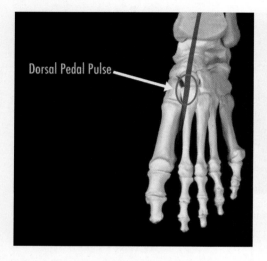

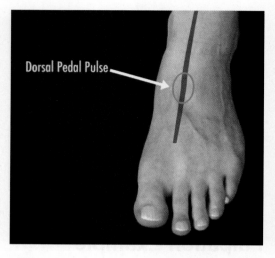

The dorsal pedal pulse is located just lateral to the extensor hallucis longus tendon where it crosses the cuneiforms.

Palpation Example

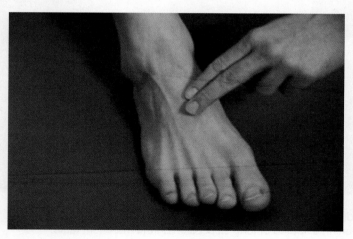

To palpate the dorsal pedal pulse,
1) Place the patient in the seated or long sit position on the treatment table.
2) Locate the tendon of extensor hallucis longus where it crosses the cuneiforms.
3) With the pads of the index and middle fingers, palpate the tendon, then move laterally just off the tendon.
4) The dorsal pedal pulse should be felt under the fingers.
5) If the pulse is not distinguishable, apply slight pressure and/or move slightly more distally.

● Extensor Digitorum Longus Tendons

Skeletal and Anatomical Landmarks

Skeletal

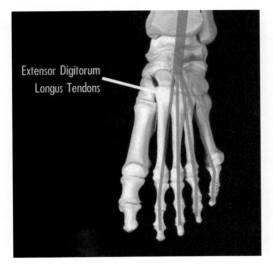

Anatomical

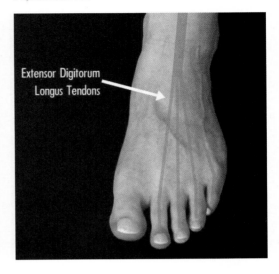

The extensor digitorum longus tendon crosses the ankle lateral to the extensor hallucis longus tendon. The tendon then splits into four slips and inserts on the 2nd and 3rd phalanges of toes 2–5.

Palpation Example

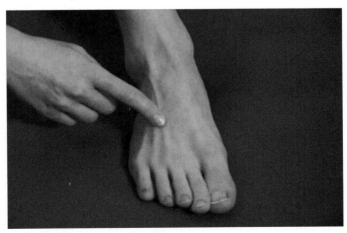

To palpate the extensor digitorum longus tendons,
1) Place the patient in a long sit position on the treatment table.
2) Ask the patient to extend the toes.
3) Locate the four tendons on the dorsum of the foot that become visible when the toes are extended.
4) The tendons merge to a common tendon that lies lateral to the anterior tibialis and extensor hallucis longus tendons as it crosses the ankle.
5) The extensor digitorum longus tendons can be palpated from the metatarsophalangeal (MTP) joints of toes 2–5 to the anterior ankle.

⦿ Extensor Hallucis Longus Tendon

Skeletal and Anatomical Landmarks

Skeletal

Anatomical

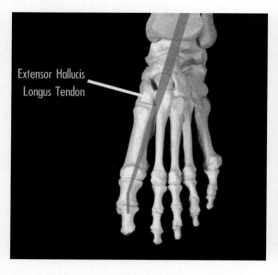

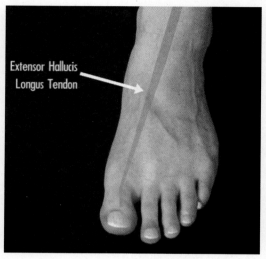

The extensor hallucis longus tendon crosses the anterior ankle just lateral to the tibialis anterior tendon. It inserts on the distal phalanx of the great toe.

Palpation Example

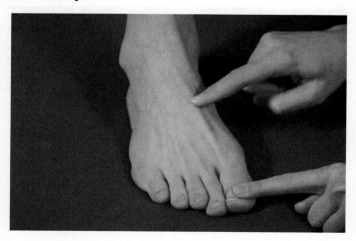

To palpate the extensor hallucis longus tendon,
1) Place the patient in a long sit position on the treatment table.
2) Ask the patient to extend the great toe against slight resistance.
3) A tendon will become visible and palpable from the phalanx of the great toe to the ankle. This tendon is the extensor hallucis longus tendon.
4) It crosses the ankle lateral to the anterior tibialis tendon and medial to the extensor digitorum longus tendon.

Flexor Digitorum Longus Tendons

Skeletal and Anatomical Landmarks

Skeletal

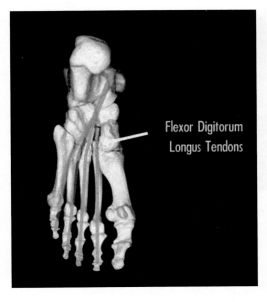

Flexor Digitorum
Longus Tendons

Anatomical

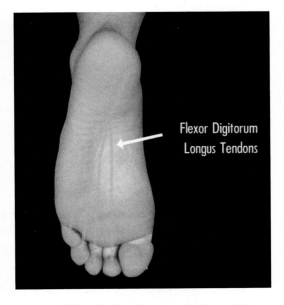

Flexor Digitorum
Longus Tendons

The flexor digitorum longus tendon runs posterior to the medial malleolus then travels through the plantar foot and attaches to the distal phalanges of toes 2–5.

Palpation Example

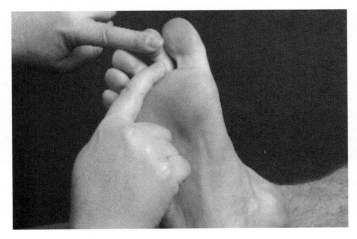

To palpate the flexor digitorum longus tendons,
1) Place the patient in the long sit position.
2) While holding the distal phalanx with one hand, ask the patient to flex the toes against slight resistance.
3) Use the index finger or thumb of your other hand to locate the tendons that become prominent at the plantar surface of the interphalangeal joints of toes 2–5.

● Flexor Hallucis Longus Tendon

Skeletal and Anatomical Landmarks

Skeletal

Anatomical

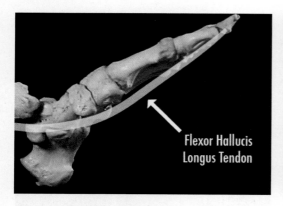

Flexor Hallucis
Longus Tendon

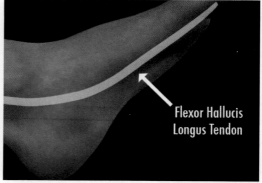

Flexor Hallucis
Longus Tendon

The flexor hallucis longus tendon crosses the ankle behind the medial malleolus and inserts on the plantar surface of the distal phalanx of the great toe.

Palpation Example

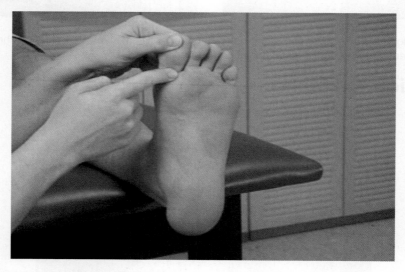

To palpate the flexor hallucis longus tendon,
1) Place the patient in a long sit position.
2) While holding the distal phalanx of the first toe, ask the patient to flex the toe against slight resistance.
3) Use the index finger or thumb of your other hand to locate the tendon that becomes prominent on the plantar surface of the proximal phalanx.

● Gastrocnemius Muscle

Skeletal and Anatomical Landmarks

Skeletal

Anatomical

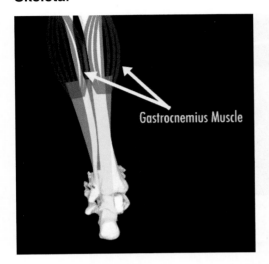

Gastrocnemius Muscle

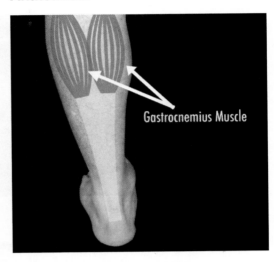

Gastrocnemius Muscle

The gastrocnemius muscle is the large calf muscle. It originates on the distal femur and inserts on the calcaneus via the Achilles tendon.

Palpation Example

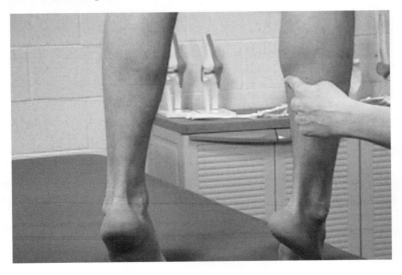

To palpate the gastrocnemius muscle,
1) Place the patient in either the prone or standing position.
2) The gastrocnemius muscle is best palpated by having the patient plantar flex against resistance or stand on the toes. This action causes the muscle to contract, which creates two distinct heads, the more prominent medial head and the lesser prominent lateral head.
3) Locate the two portions of the muscle that appear as an upside down heart on the posterior lower leg.

◉ Heads of the Metatarsals

Skeletal and Anatomical Landmarks

Skeletal

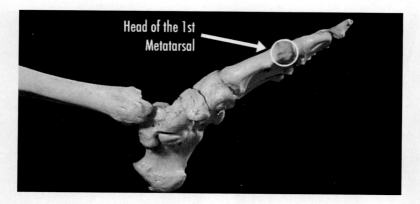

Head of the 1st
Metatarsal

Anatomical

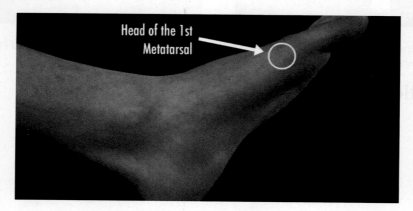

Head of the 1st
Metatarsal

The head of the metatarsal is the distal end of the metatarsal.

Palpation Example

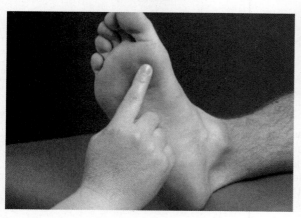

To palpate the head of each metatarsal,
1) Place the patient in a long sit position on the treatment table.
2) Locate what is commonly referred to as the ball of the foot.
3) The head of the metatarsal is the proximal portion of that area. Using your thumb, one finger, or by holding the metatarsal head between your thumb and index finger, palpate the full circumference of the bone.

◉ Head of the Talus

Skeletal and Anatomical Landmarks

Skeletal

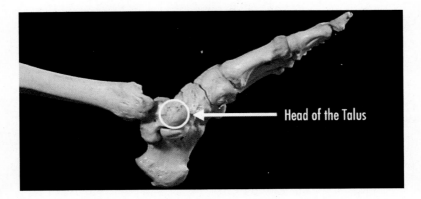

Head of the Talus

Anatomical

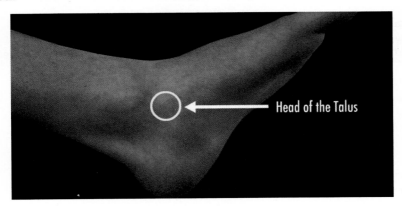

Head of the Talus

The head of the talus is the distal portion of the talus that articulates with the navicular bone. It is easily palpable on the medial aspect of the foot.

Palpation Example

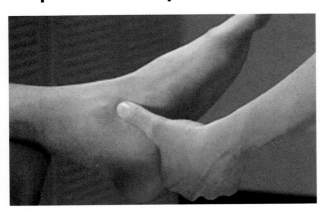

To palpate the head of the talus,
1) Place the patient in a seated position at the end of the treatment table.
2) Locate the navicular tubercle, then
3) Move half the distance between the navicular tubercle and the medial malleolus.
4) The small bony protrusion felt at that location is the head of the talus.

Invert and Evert Foot

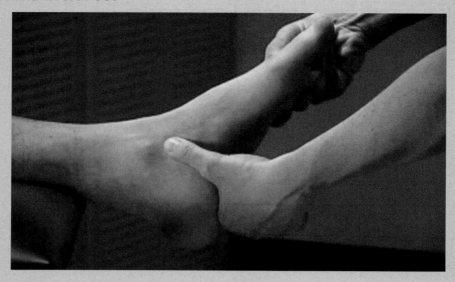

To verify that you are on the head of the talus,
1) Passively invert and evert the foot while palpating the head of the talus.
2) The head of the talus will protrude and retract as the foot is everted and inverted, respectively.

◉ Lateral Malleolus

Skeletal and Anatomical Landmarks

Skeletal

Anatomical

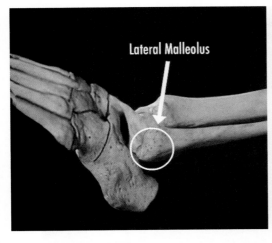

Lateral Malleolus

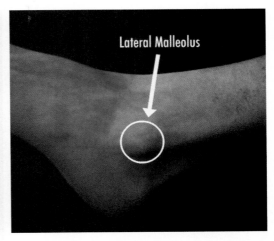

Lateral Malleolus

The lateral malleolus is the large protruding bone on the outside of the ankle. It is the distal end of the fibula.

Palpation Example

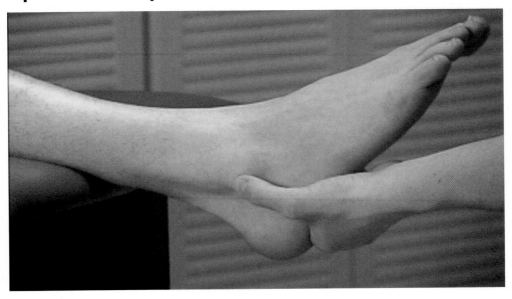

To palpate the lateral malleolus,
1) Place the patient in a seated position at the end of the treatment table or in a long sit position on the treatment table.
2) The lateral malleolus is easily distinguishable since it is the large protruding bone on the outside of the ankle.
3) Locate the bone and palpate over its full surface.

⊙ Long Plantar Ligament

Skeletal and Anatomical Landmarks

Skeletal   **Anatomical**

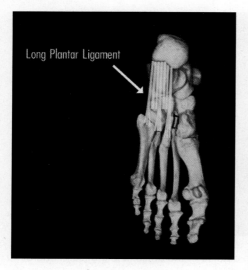
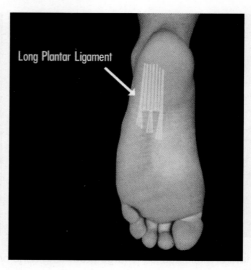

The long plantar ligament originates on the plantar surface of the calcaneus and inserts on the cuboid and bases of the lateral metatarsals.

Palpation Example

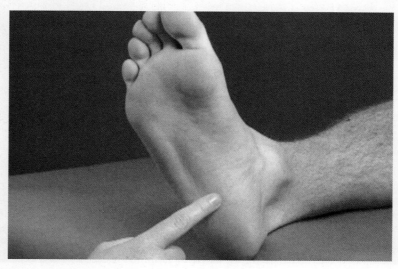

To palpate the long plantar ligament,
1) Place the patient in a long sit position on the treatment table.
2) Locate the deeper, thick band that lies between the calcaneus and cuboid/metatarsal bases.
3) Using your thumb or fingers, palpate the ligament over its full length.

⦿ Medial Malleolus

Skeletal and Anatomical Landmarks

Skeletal   **Anatomical**

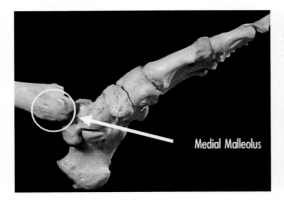
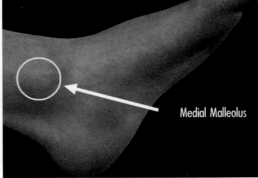

The medial malleolus is the distal end of the tibia. It is the large bony protrusion on the inside of the ankle.

Palpation Example

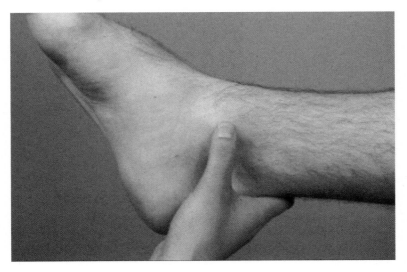

To palpate the medial malleolus,
1) Place the patient in a seated position at the end of the treatment table or in a long sit position on the treatment table.
2) The medial malleolus is easily distinguishable since it is the large protruding bone on the inside of the ankle.
3) Locate the bone and palpate over its full surface.

⦿ Medial Tubercle of the Calcaneus

Skeletal and Anatomical Landmarks

Skeletal   **Anatomical**

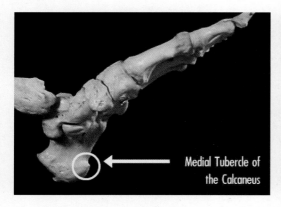   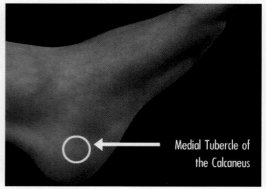

The medial calcaneal tubercle is the protrusion of bone located on the medial plantar aspect of the foot. It serves as the attachment for the plantar fascia.

Palpation Example

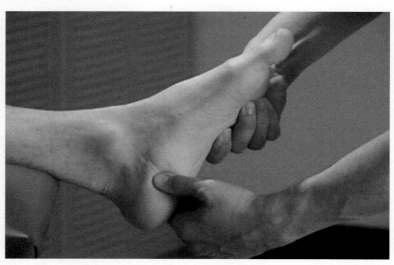

To palpate the medial tubercle of the calcaneus,
1) Place the patient in a seated position at the end of the treatment table or in a long sit position on the treatment table.
2) Start at the midfoot and palpate along the medial longitudinal arch toward the heel, staying along the imaginary line where the more calloused plantar aspect of the foot meets the softer skin of the side of the foot.
3) The medial calcaneal tubercle is felt as a harder bony "block" at the proximal end of the arch, about one-third of the way onto the "heel pad."

TIP

Tender Area

The area of the medial calcaneal tubercle is tender, allowing the evaluator to recognize when the landmark has been located.

Imaginary Line

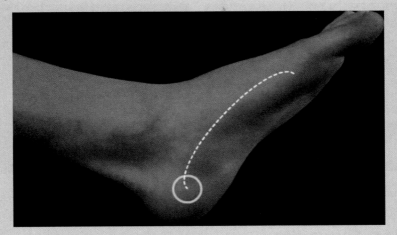

The medial calcaneal tubercle is located at the proximal end of the medial longitudinal arch, along the imaginary line where the more calloused plantar aspect of the foot meets the softer skin of the side of the foot.

◉ Medial Tubercle of the Talus

Skeletal and Anatomical Landmarks

Skeletal   **Anatomical**

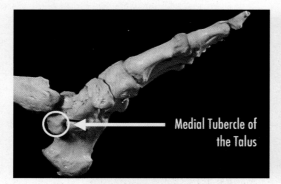

Medial Tubercle of
the Talus

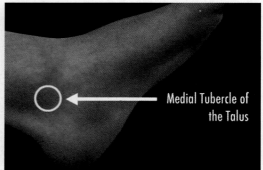

Medial Tubercle of
the Talus

The medial tubercle of the talus is located just distal and posterior to the distal tip of the medial malleolus.

Palpation Example

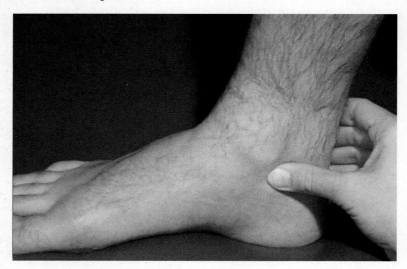

To palpate the medial tubercle of the talus,
1) Place the patient in a seated position at the end of the treatment table or in a long sit position on the treatment table.
2) Locate the medial malleolus, then
3) Move inferiorly just off the malleolus and posteriorly approximately one finger width.
4) The tubercle can be felt as a tiny ball or drop-off and tends to be quite tender when palpated.

● Metatarsals

Skeletal and Anatomical Landmarks

Skeletal

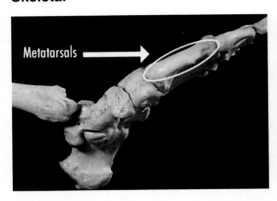

Anatomical

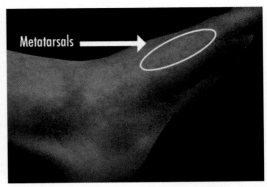

The metatarsals are the long bones in the foot, distal to the cuneiforms and cuboid and proximal to the toes.

Palpation Example

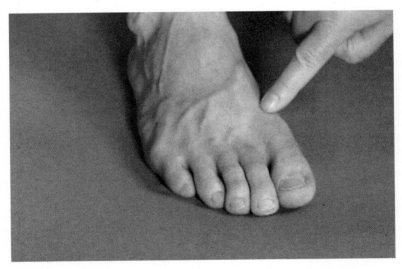

To palpate the metatarsals,
1) Place the patient in a seated position at the end of the treatment table or in a long sit position on the treatment table.
2) Locate the long bones on the dorsum of the foot.
3) They are directly proximal to each toe and extend one-half to two-thirds of the way to the ankle.

Metatarsophalangeal Joints

Skeletal and Anatomical Landmarks

Skeletal

Anatomical

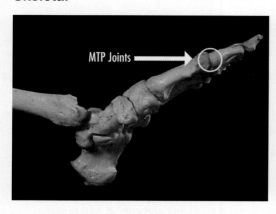

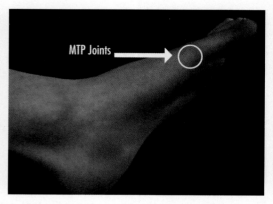

The metatarsophalangeal (MTP) joints are the joints between the foot and the toes.

Palpation Example

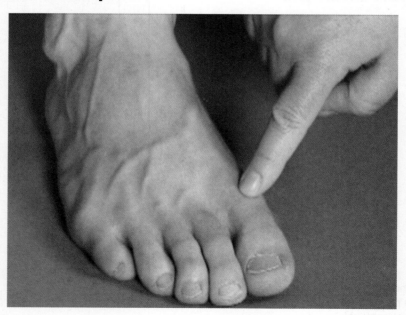

To palpate the MTP joints,
1) Place the patient in a seated position on the end of the treatment table or in a long sit position on the treatment table.
2) Locate what is commonly referred to as the balls of the foot or the first knuckles where the toes meet the foot.
3) The MTP joints lie in the center of those areas.

◉ Navicular Tubercle

Skeletal and Anatomical Landmarks

Skeletal   **Anatomical**

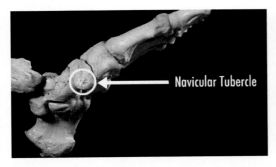 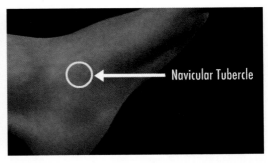

The navicular tubercle is the most prominent bone on the medial aspect of the foot at about the midpoint of the medial longitudinal arch.

Palpation Example

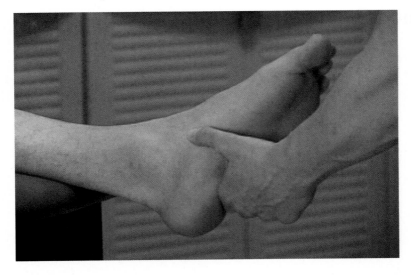

To palpate the navicular tubercle,
1) Place the patient in a seated position at the end of the treatment table or in a long sit position on the treatment table.
2) Locate the navicular tubercle by running your finger along the medial aspect of the foot near the midpoint of the medial longitudinal arch.
3) The navicular tubercle is typically the most prominent bone in that region.

TIP

Verifying the Landmark
To verify that you are on the navicular tubercle, palpate under the bone to see if it has a large shelflike drop-off. It if does, it is the navicular tubercle rather than the first cuneiform.

◉ Peroneal Tubercle

Skeletal and Anatomical Landmarks

Skeletal   **Anatomical**

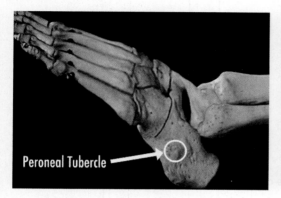

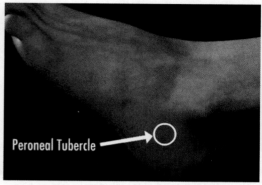

The peroneal tubercle is a small protrusion on the lateral calcaneus, distal to the malleolus. The peroneus brevis and longus tendons split at this point as they progress toward their insertion points.

Palpation Example

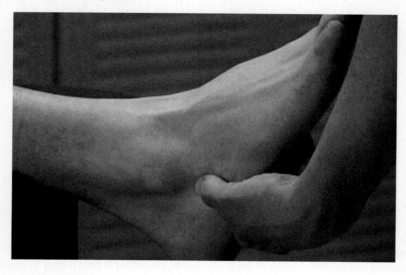

To palpate the peroneal tubercle,
1) Place the patient in a seated position at the end of the treatment table or in a long sit position on the treatment table.
2) Locate the lateral malleolus then move distally approximately two finger widths and slightly anteriorly.
3) The peroneal tubercle can be felt as a small bump.
4) The split in the peroneus (fibularis) longus and brevis tendons may also be visible or palpable at this point.

◉ Peroneus (Fibularis) Brevis Tendon

Skeletal and Anatomical Landmarks

Skeletal

Anatomical

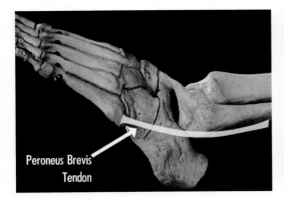

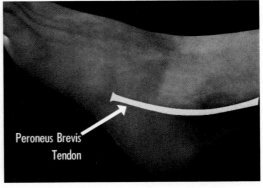

The peroneus (fibularis) brevis tendon runs behind the lateral malleolus and attaches to the posterior aspect of the base of the fifth metatarsal.

Palpation Example

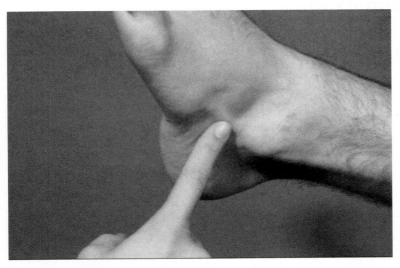

To palpate the peroneus (fibularis) brevis tendon,
1) Place the patient in a seated position at the end of the treatment table or in a long sit position on the treatment table.
2) Ask the patient to slightly evert the foot against gentle resistance.
3) Locate the tendon that should be visible and palpable superior and posterior to the lateral malleolus all the way to the base of the fifth metatarsal.

◉ Peroneus (Fibularis) Longus Tendon

Skeletal and Anatomical Landmarks

Skeletal   **Anatomical**

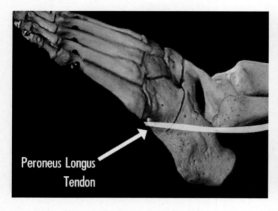

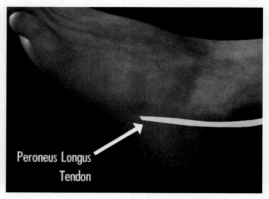

The peroneus (fibularis) longus tendon runs behind the lateral malleolus. The peroneus longus and brevis tendons split apart near the peroneal tubercle. The peroneus longus tendon passes just proximal to the base of the 5th metatarsal as it dives down to the plantar aspect of the foot.

Palpation Example

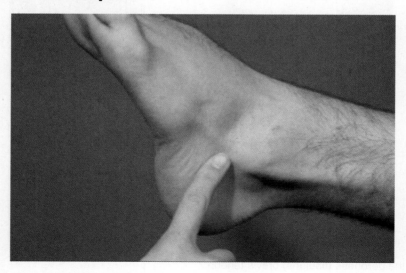

To palpate the peroneus (fibularis) longus tendon,
1) Place the patient in a seated position at the end of the treatment table or in a long sit position on the treatment table.
2) Ask the patient to slightly evert the foot against gentle resistance.
3) Locate the tendon that should be visible and palpable superior and posterior to the lateral malleolus then distal to the lateral malleolus to the peroneal tubercle.
4) The tendon runs straighter toward the bottom of the foot than does the peroneus brevis.
5) It will disappear near the peroneal tubercle as it "dives" deep to go under the foot.

● Peroneus (Fibularis) Tertius Tendon

Skeletal and Anatomical Landmarks

Skeletal

Anatomical

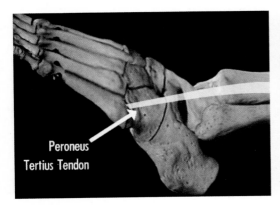
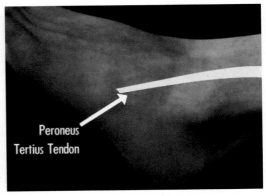

The peroneus (fibularis) tertius tendon crosses the ankle anterior to the lateral malleolus and inserts on the superior surface of the styloid process.

Palpation Example

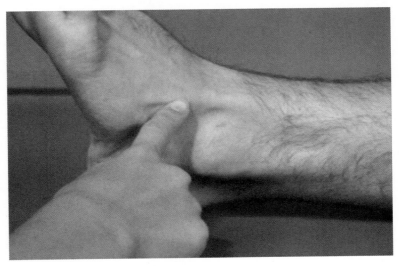

To palpate the peroneus (fibularis) tertius tendon,
1) Place the patient in a seated position at the end of the treatment table or in a long sit position on the treatment table.
2) Ask the patient to evert and slightly dorsiflex the foot against gentle resistance.
3) Locate the tendon that can be palpated (and often visualized) as it passes anterior to the lateral malleolus, runs with the extensor digitorum longus tendon, then diverts off laterally to insert on the styloid process.

● Phalanges (Foot)

Skeletal and Anatomical Landmarks

Skeletal   **Anatomical**

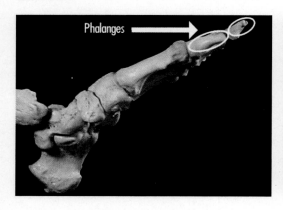   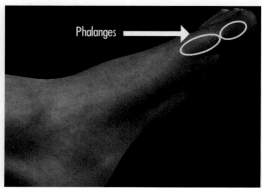

The phalanges are the bones of the toes.

Palpation Example

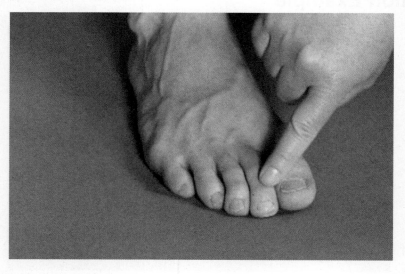

To palpate the phalanges of the foot,
1) Place the patient in a seated position at the end of the treatment table.
2) Locate each segment of the toes, remembering there are only two phalanges in the great toe and three in each of the others.
3) The phalanges can be palpated with a single finger or by gently pinching the bones between your thumb and fingers.

● Plantar Fascia

Skeletal and Anatomical Landmarks

Skeletal | **Anatomical**

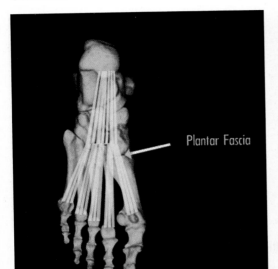

Plantar Fascia

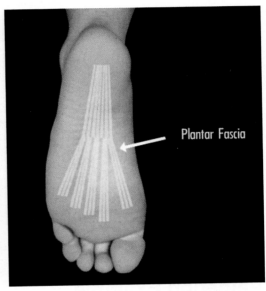

Plantar Fascia

The plantar fascia originates at the medial calcaneal tubercle. It extends over the entire sole of the foot then inserts near the metatarsal heads.

Palpation Example

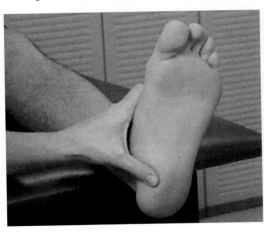

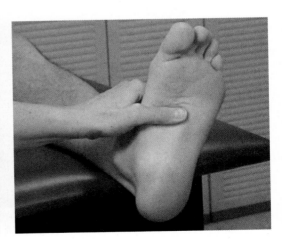

To palpate the plantar fascia,
1) Place the patient in a long sit position on the treatment table.
2) Starting at the plantar surface of the medial tubercle of the calcaneus, locate the fibrous band at the bottom of the foot (the plantar fascia).
3) Follow the fibrous band through the arch of the foot to the metatarsal heads.

◉ Posterior Talofibular Ligament

Skeletal and Anatomical Landmarks

Skeletal   **Anatomical**

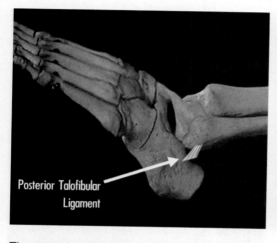

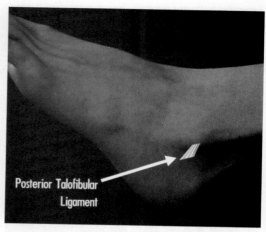

The posterior talofibular ligament originates from the back of the mid lateral malleolus and runs almost horizontally to the posterior talus.

Palpation Example

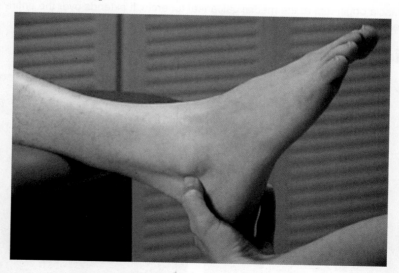

To palpate the posterior talofibular (PTF) ligament,
1) Place the patient in a seated position at the end of the treatment table or in a long sit position on the treatment table.
2) Locate the lateral malleolus, then
3) Move posteriorly off the back of the mid portion of the malleolus.
4) The ligament lies in the groove between the malleolus and the talus and can be felt as a small band.

● Posterior Tibial Pulse

Skeletal and Anatomical Landmarks

Skeletal

Anatomical

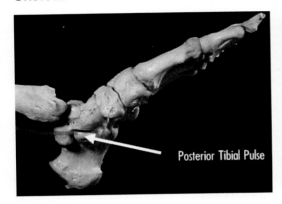

Posterior Tibial Pulse

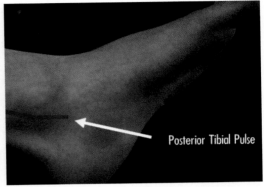

Posterior Tibial Pulse

The posterior tibial artery passes behind the medial malleolus where it is easily palpable.

Palpation Example

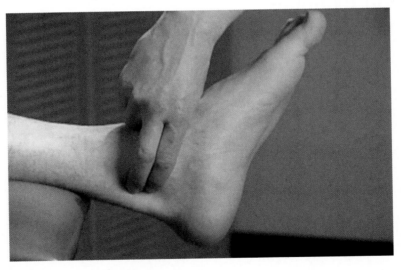

To palpate the posterior tibial pulse,
1) Place the patient in a seated position at the end of the treatment table.
2) Locate the medial malleolus, then
3) Slide your fingers posteriorly into the groove behind the malleolus.
4) Press in gently against the bone with 2–3 fingers to feel the pulse.

◉ Posterior Tibiofibular Ligament

Skeletal and Anatomical Landmarks

Skeletal

Anatomical

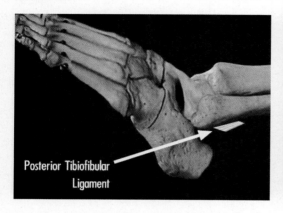

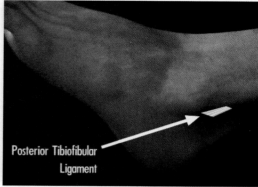

The posterior tibiofibular ligament orginates at the back of the superior portion of the lateral malleolus and inserts on the distal posterior-lateral tibia.

Palpation Example

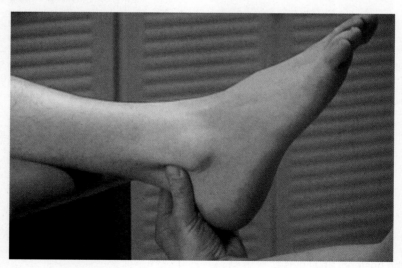

To palpate the posterior tibiofibular ligament,
1) Place the patient in a seated position at the end of the treatment table or in a long sit position on the treatment table.
2) Locate the lateral malleolus, then
3) Move 2–3 finger widths proximally along the fibular shaft and posteriorly into the deeper groove beside the fibula.
4) Palpate with a single digit or pinch the front and back of the fibula between your thumb and fingers and move in a short superior-inferior motion along the shaft.
5) The ligament may not be distinguishable but pain in the area may be experienced if the ligament is injured.

● Proximal Interphalangeal Joints (Foot)

Skeletal and Anatomical Landmarks

Skeletal

Anatomical

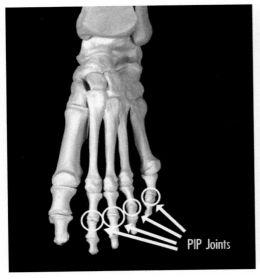
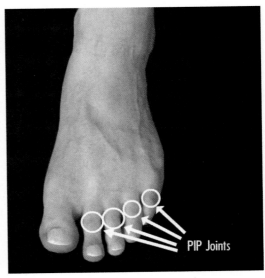

The proximal interphalangeal (PIP) joint is the most proximal joint of the two joints in toes 2–5.

Palpation Example

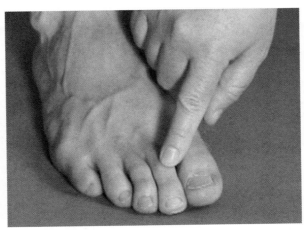

To palpate the PIP joints of the foot,
1) Place the patient in a seated position at the end of the treatment table.
2) Locate the most proximal joint of the two interphalangeal joints of toes 2–5.
3) The joints can be palpated with a single finger or by gently pinching the joints between your thumb and fingers.

◉ Sesamoid Bones

Skeletal and Anatomical Landmarks

Skeletal   **Anatomical**

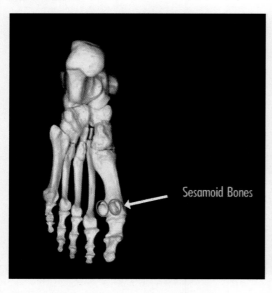
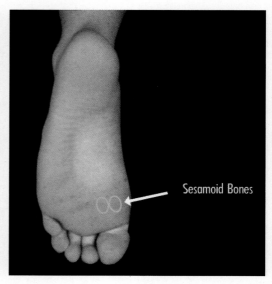

The sesamoid bones lie on the plantar aspect of the 1st metatarsal head, just proximal to the MP joint.

Palpation Example

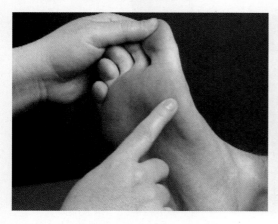
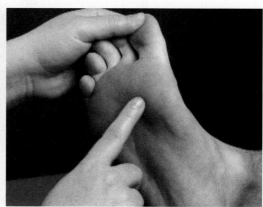

To palpate the sesamoid bones of the foot,
1) Place the patient in a long sit position on the treatment table.
2) The sesamoid bones are located just proximal to the MTP joint line of the first toe (big toe).
3) Locate the MTP joint line, then
4) Move proximally and both medially and laterally from the metatarsal head's midline.
5) Both sesamoid bones are felt as small bony protrusions, with the medial sesamoid being more prominent.
6) The medial sesamoid bone also tends to lie slightly more proximally than the lateral one.
   Both are tender to palpate.

◉ Shaft of the Fibula

Skeletal and Anatomical Landmarks

Skeletal

Anatomical

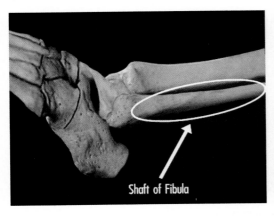

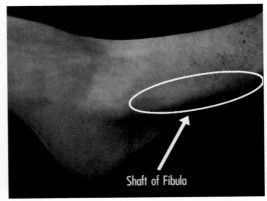

The shaft of the fibula is the long portion of the bone between the lateral malleolus and the fibular head.

Palpation Example

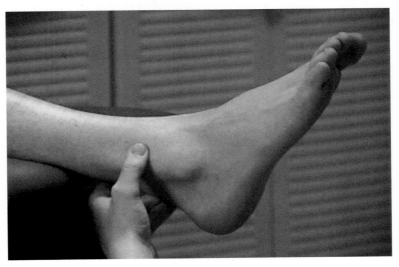

To palpate the shaft of the fibula,
1) Place the patient in a seated position at the end of the treatment table or in a long sit position on the treatment table.
2) The shaft of the fibula is best palpated just superior to the lateral malleolus.
3) Locate the lateral malleolus, then follow the fibula superiorly for several inches.

● Shaft of the Tibia

Skeletal and Anatomical Landmarks

Skeletal

Anatomical

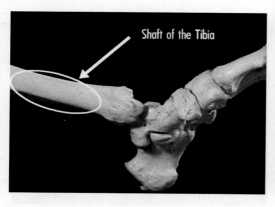

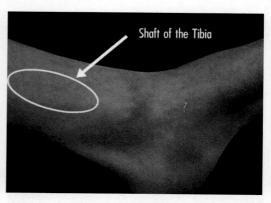

The shaft of the tibia is commonly referred to as the shin bone.

Palpation Example

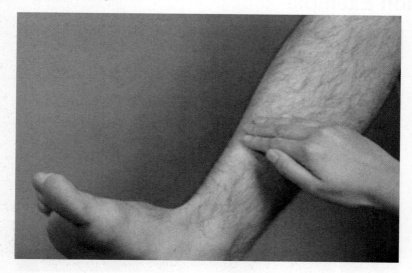

To palpate the shaft of the tibia,

1) Place the patient in a seated position at the end of the treatment table or in a long sit position on the treatment table.
2) Locate the bone that is commonly referred to as the shin bone on the anterior lower leg.
3) Palpate the full length of the bone.

● Sinus Tarsi

Skeletal and Anatomical Landmarks

Skeletal   **Anatomical**

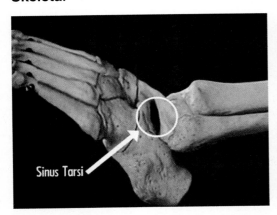 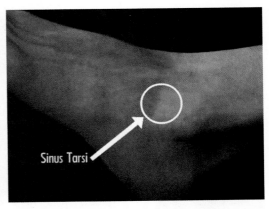

The sinus tarsi is the large indentation on the lateral ankle, anterior to the lateral malleolus.

Palpation Example

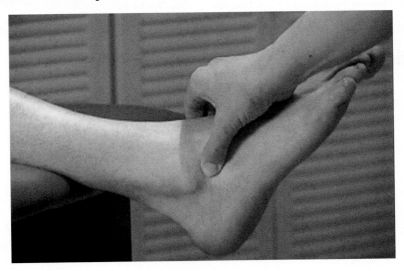

To palpate the sinus tarsi,
1) Place the patient in a seated position at the end of the treatment table or in a long sit position on the treatment table.
2) Locate the lateral malleolus, then
3) Move anteriorly to the large indentation.
4) This indentation is the sinus tarsi.

Soleus Muscle

Skeletal and Anatomical Landmarks

Skeletal   **Anatomical**

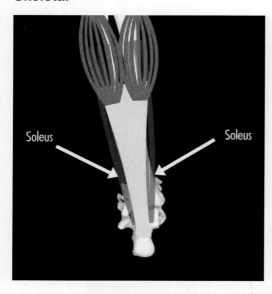
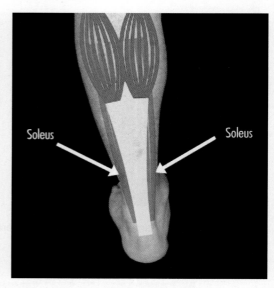

The soleus muscle lies deep to the gastrocnemius and extends more distally than the gastrocnemius.

Palpation Example

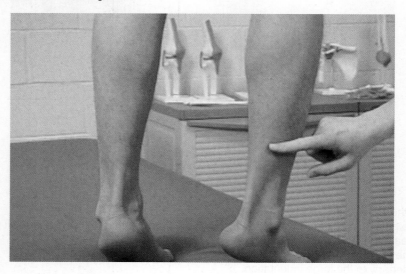

To palpate the soleus muscle,
1) Place the patient in a seated position at the end of the treatment table or standing.
2) Ask the patient to plantar flex against gentle resistance (or stand on the toes).
3) Locate the soleus by palpating the muscle that becomes prominent distal to the lateral head of the gastrocnemius, along the posterior lateral aspect of the leg.

● Spring Ligament

Skeletal and Anatomical Landmarks

Skeletal

Anatomical

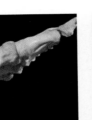

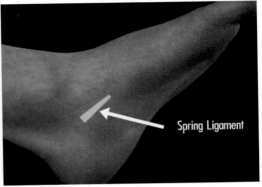

The plantar calcaneonavicular ligament (or spring ligament) runs from the plantar surface of the navicular to the anterior border of the sustentaculum tali.

Palpation Example

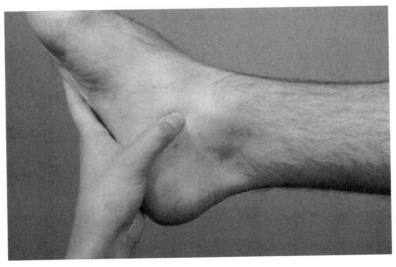

To palpate the spring ligament,
1) Place the patient in a seated position at the end of the treatment table.
2) Locate the navicular tubercle, then
3) Move to its inferior edge, palpating under the bone.
4) The spring ligament can be palpated as a small band from the plantar surface of the navicular tubercle to the sustentaculum tali (about 1–2 inches).

⦿ Sustentaculum Tali

Skeletal and Anatomical Landmarks

Skeletal

Anatomical

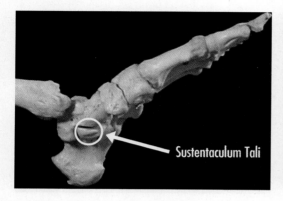

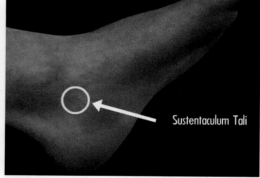

The sustentaculum tali is a larger, shelflike protrusion of bone on the medial calcaneus. It lies distal to the medial malleolus and serves as an attachment for the spring ligament.

Palpation Example

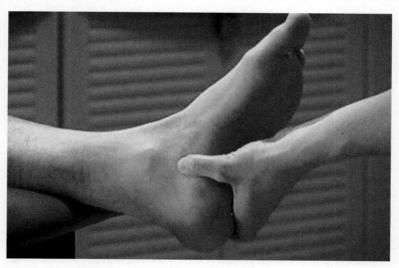

To palpate the sustentaculum tali,
1) Place the patient in a seated position at the end of the treatment table or in a long sit position on the treatment table.
2) Using your thumb, locate the medial malleolus then
3) Move directly inferiorly 1–1½ finger widths until a bony drop-off is felt.
4) Pull back up into the bony drop-off.
5) This bone is the sustentaculum tali and is often tender to palpate.

Tibialis Anterior Tendon

Skeletal and Anatomical Landmarks

Skeletal

Anatomical

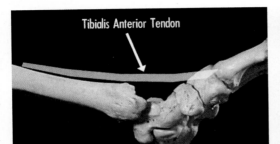

Tibialis Anterior Tendon

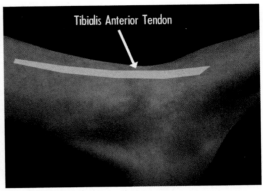

Tibialis Anterior Tendon

The tibialis anterior tendon is the large tendon that crosses the anterior ankle. It runs from the superior lateral ankle to medial foot and is responsible for dorsiflexing and inverting the foot.

Palpation Example

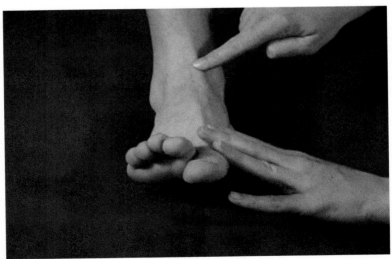

To palpate the tibialis anterior tendon,
1) Place the patient in a seated position at the end of the treatment table.
2) Ask the patient to dorsiflex and invert the foot (against resistance if possible).
3) The tibialis anterior tendon becomes visible and palpable on the anterior ankle as it crosses from superior lateral ankle to the medial foot.
4) The tendon can be palpated with a single finger or by gently pinching the tendon between your thumb and fingers.

◉ Tibialis Posterior Tendon

Skeletal and Anatomical Landmarks

Skeletal   **Anatomical**

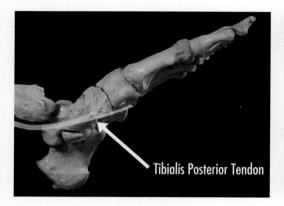

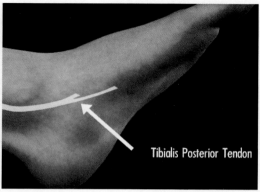

The tibialis posterior tendon runs posterior to the medial malleolus then extends distally to the plantar aspect of the foot where it attaches on several metatarsal bases and tarsal bones.

Palpation Example

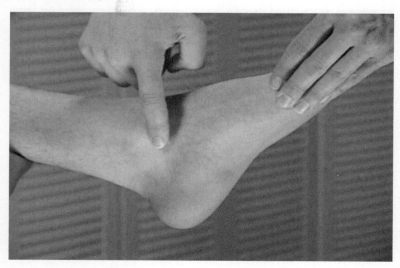

To palpate the tibialis posterior tendon,
1) Place the patient in a seated position at the end of the treatment table.
2) The tibialis posterior tendon can be palpated posterior to the medial malleolus but is most consistently palpable distal to the malleolus.
3) Ask the patient to slightly invert the foot against resistance.
4) Locate the tendon that becomes prominent just distal and anterior to the malleolus.
5) The tendon can be palpated for about 1–2 inches and can sometimes be mistaken for a bony prominence due to its firmness when contracted.